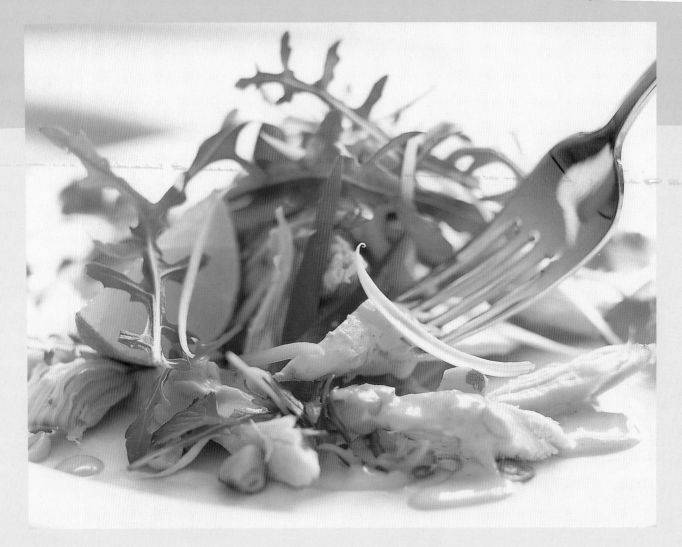

GREAT HEALTHY FOOD™
FOR
STRONG BONES

FIONA HUNTER & EMMA-LEE GOW

FIREFLY BOOKS

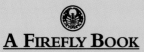

A FIREFLY BOOK

Published by Firefly Books Ltd, 2003

First edition

National Library of Canada Cataloguing in Publication Data
Hunter, Fiona
Great healthy food for strong bones / Fiona Hunter, Emma-Lee Gow.
Includes index.
ISBN 1-55297-652-1
1. High-calcium diet—Recipes. I. Gow, Emma-Lee II. Title.
RM237.56.H87 2002   641.5′632
C2002-902715-2

Publisher Cataloging-in-Publication Data (U.S.)
Hunter, Fiona.
Great Healthy Food for Strong Bones / Fiona Hunter & Emma-Lee Gow. — 1st ed.
[128] p. : col. photos. ; cm.
Includes index.
Summary: Recipes for dishes high in calcium to help prevent osteoporosis.
ISBN 1-55297-652-1 (pbk.)
1. High-calcium diet – Recipes.
2. Osteoporosis – Prevention. I. Gow, Emma-Lee. II. Title.
641.5/63 dc 21   RM237.56.H86   2003

Managing Editor Becky Alexander
Editor Jessica Hughes
Designer Justin Ford
Photography David Murray, Jules Selmes
Food Stylist Clare Lewis

Published in the United States by
Firefly Books (U.S.) Inc.
P.O. Box 1338, Ellicott Station
Buffalo, New York 14205

Published in Canada by
Firefly Books Ltd.
3680 Victoria Park Avenue
Toronto, Ontario M3H 3K1

Created and produced by
Carroll & Brown Publishers Limited
20 Lonsdale Road, London NW6 6RD

Reproduced by Colourscan, Singapore
Printed in Italy

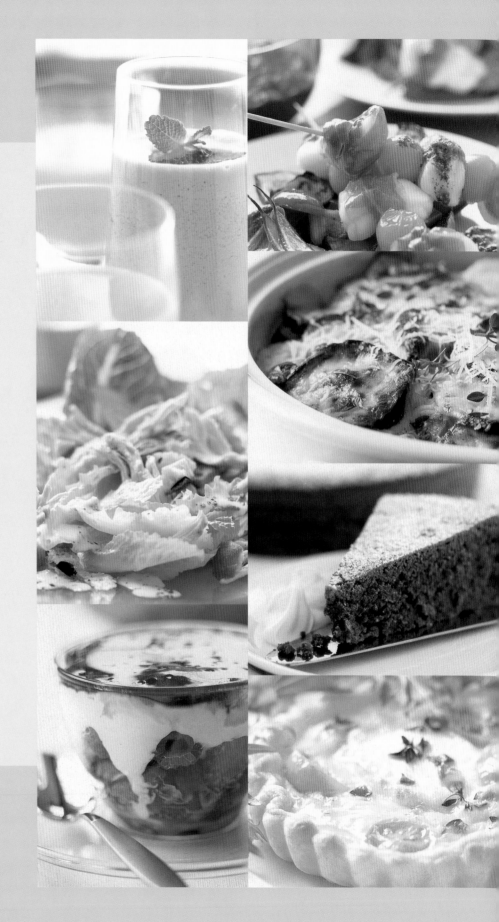

Contents

Introduction

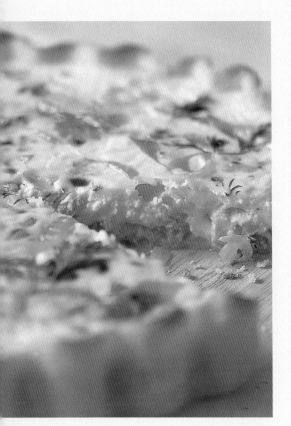

One of the most important ways in which we can develop and maintain strong bones is through a healthy diet; choosing a healthy, well-balanced and varied diet that includes foods from each of the main food groups will help ensure a good intake of vitamins and minerals, espcially calcium, which is essential for good bone health. Building strong bones when we are young and helping to reduce the effects of bone-density loss as we get older means that we can alleviate many of the symptoms of osteoporosis. This book features a wide variety of delicious recipes that have been devised to help you develop a diet that is great for strong, healthy bones and that will appeal to all the family. The recipes will also fit easily into your lifestyle, as the dishes are easy to prepare and all the ingredients are readily available in supermarkets.

Diet and Osteoporosis

A poor diet will increase the risk of osteoporosis (also known as brittle bone disease) later in life. Osteoporosis affects 1 in 3 women and 1 in 12 men during their lifetimes. Bones are made up of a thick outer shell with a strong, dense inner mesh that has a honeycomblike structure. A good calcium intake is vital because this gives the bones their strength and rigidity. As bone becomes old, it is removed by the body and replaced with new bone—it has been calculated that adults replace their entire skeletons every 7 to 10 years. Calcium, therefore, gets deposited and withdrawn from the skeleton on a daily basis. As we get older, this renewal process slows down and bone-density loss increases. When this happens, the holes in the bone's inner mesh gradually become bigger and the bones become more fragile and, therefore, more likely to fracture or break—this is known as osteoporosis. However, by maximizing bone mass early in life and by maintaining a healthy diet, we can reduce the effects of this process.

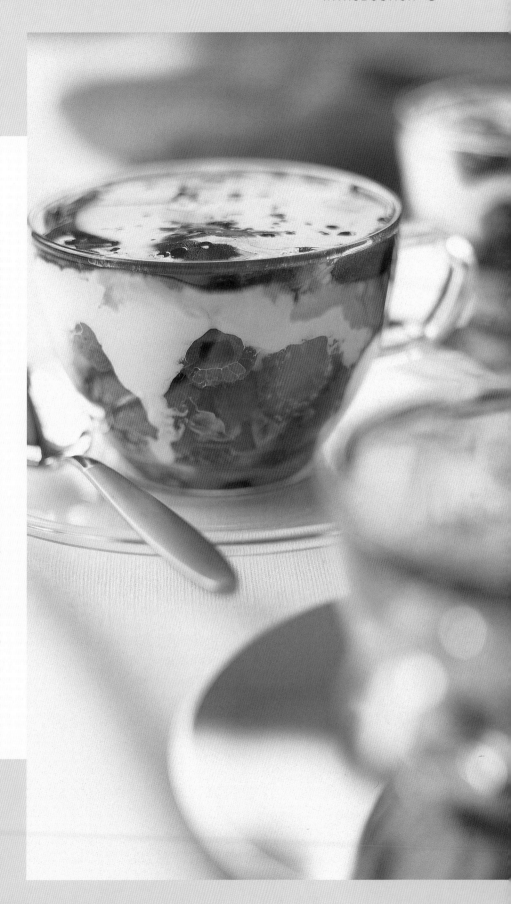

CALCIUM FOR EVERYONE

It's never too early or too late to begin eating for strong bones. A good calcium intake during childhood, adolescence, and early adulthood, while the bones are still growing, will help to protect your bones throughout life. By the age of 25, your bones have reached their maximum potential strength, so it is important to invest in them in the early years. As we move into later life, maintaining a calcium-rich diet is equally important in order to reduce the effects of bone loss. Bone density begins to decrease around age 35, so it is essential to maintain a bone-friendly diet throughout life.

Pregnant women need a good calcium intake to provide for the calcium needs of their babies. People on low-fat diets also need to ensure they are not missing out on calcium-rich foods such as dairy products. It is important to remember that low-

THE OSTEOPOROSIS SOCIETY OF CANADA

The OSC is a national organization serving people who have, or are at risk for, osteoporosis. A registered charity, the OSC works to educate, empower and support individuals and communities in the prevention and treatment of osteoporosis. Its bilingual toll-free information line offers a wide variety of free publications, programs and referrals to self-help groups and community resources. For more information visit www.osteoporosis.ca

THE NATIONAL OSTEOPOROSIS FOUNDATION

The NOF is major resource in the USA for individuals, organizations and professionals seeking information on osteoporosis. To raise awareness of the causes of bone-related diseases and improve prevention, diagnosis and treatment, it publishes a variety of educational materials. For more information visit www.nof.org

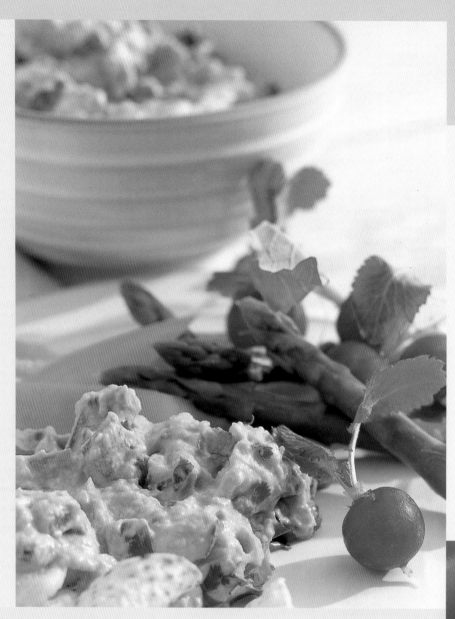

RECOMMENDED DAILY ALLOWANCES OF CALCIUM

Age	Daily intake*	Number of servings**
Children, 4–8 years	800 mg	2–3
Children, 9–13 years	1300 mg	4
Teenagers, 14–18 years	1300-1400 mg	4
Men and women, 19–50 years	1000 mg	3–4
Men and women, 51–70 years	1000 mg	3–4
Men and women, 51–70 years (high risk)	1200 mg	3–4
Men and women, 70 years and over	1200 mg	3–4
Pregnant or breastfeeding women	1000 mg	3–4

* These figures represent high averages of the OSC and NOF recommended daily allowances of calcium.

** 1 serving = 1 glass of milk, ⅔ cup (150 ml) yogurt or ¼ cup (50 ml) hard full-fat cheese.

A HEALTHY LIFESTYLE

As well as a bone-friendly diet, there are other ways in which we can improve bone strength. Weight-bearing exercise—for example, walking, jogging, tennis, or aerobics—improves bone density, and balance exercises, such as yoga, reduce the risk of falling—active people have 20–45 percent less risk of fracture. Exercise such as swimming and cycling is good for overall fitness, but is of no benefit to the bones. Also, giving up smoking is vital for strong bones because it damages the cells that make new bone.

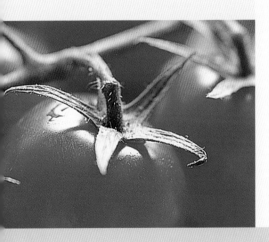

fat dairy products can still be a good source of calcium because when fat is removed to make reduced or low-fat products, the calcium remains (in fact, ounce for ounce, skim milk contains slightly more calcium than whole milk). This is especially important for teenage girls, who are more likely to embark on low-fat diets at a time when good calcium intake is vital.

BONE-FRIENDLY FOODS

As part of a diet for strong bones, and for your health in general, you need to eat a healthy, well-balanced and varied diet that includes at least 5 servings of fruit and/or vegetables a day, plenty of whole-grain cereals, and not too much sugar or fat. The following vitamins and minerals are particularly good for strong bones.

Calcium This is the most vital mineral for strong bones. Calcium is also essential for blood clotting, muscle contraction, and nerve function and, if we don't take in enough, the body uses the calcium in the bones to supply the muscles, heart, and nerves. In the average American diet, milk and other dairy products provide over 50 percent of dietary calcium, but it is also found in beans and legumes, canned fish that is eaten along with its bones—for example salmon and sardines—some green vegetables, such as spinach and broccoli, and nuts and fruit.

Vitamin D This is vital for the absorption of calcium and is produced when the skin is exposed to sunlight. About 15–20 minutes of sunlight a day on the face and arms during the summer months enables the body to store enough vitamin D to last the rest of the year. Most people obtain sufficient vitamin D in this way, but some groups, such as the elderly, housebound, or people who wear clothes that cover most of their bodies, may have insufficient vitamin D. Good food sources of vitamin D are oil-rich fish, egg yolks, liver, and margarine.

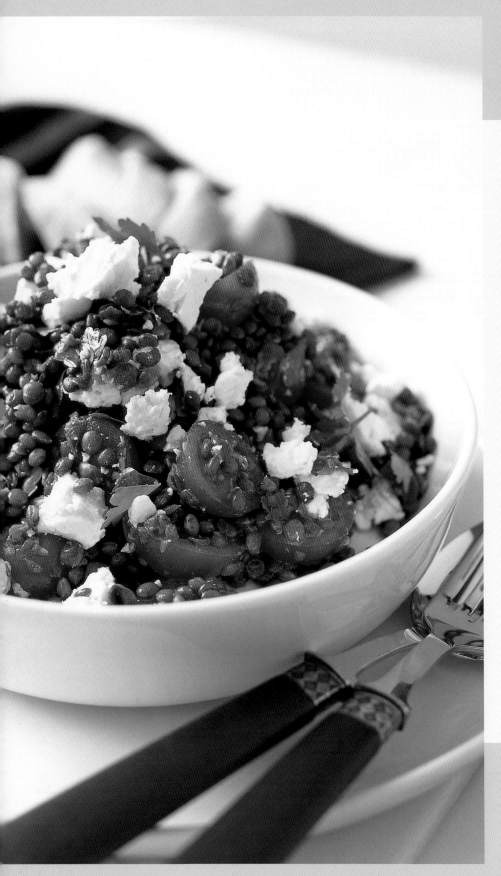

Magnesium Recent studies suggest that magnesium has an important role to play in helping to keep our bones healthy. Good sources of magnesium include Brazil nuts, sunflower seeds, sesame seeds, bananas, pine nuts, cashew nuts, and dark green leafy vegetables, such as spinach and watercress.

Vitamin K Studies have found that women who have a good intake of vitamin K have denser bones and fewer hip fractures. Foods rich in vitamin K include curly kale, broccoli, and spinach.

Be Careful With . . .

Protein High intakes of protein increase the excretion of calcium in the urine. For most people, however, protein intakes are not high enough to give cause for concern, but it could be a problem if you take protein supplements or follow a high-protein, weight-reducing diet.

Salt High sodium (salt) intake can also increase the loss of calcium in the urine. Over three-quarters of the sodium in our diet comes from processed foods, so the simplest way to reduce sodium intake is to eat fewer processed foods. Food with less salt may initially taste bland, but by gradually reducing the amount of salt you eat, the tastebuds will adapt as the salt receptors on the tongue become more sensitive. Try using other flavorings such as herbs and spices, lemon, or mustard.

Caffeine High intakes of caffeine can reduce absorption of calcium—each cup of coffee prevents the absorption of 6 mg of calcium, which is the amount you would get from 1 teaspoon (5 ml) of milk. The effect of caffeine is relatively small, but people with very high intakes should cut back.

Alcohol Excessive intakes of alcohol can damage the cells that make new bone. If you drink, stay within the recommended guidelines (up to 2 alcoholic drinks a day for men and up to 1 alcoholic drink a day for women).

Carbonated drinks Phosphate, in the form of phosphoric acid, is used as a preservative in most canned carbonated drinks. When phosphorus levels exceed calcium levels in the blood, the body responds by stimulating bone breakdown to release calcium into the blood. Although there is no hard scientific evidence to show a detrimental effect on bone health, it is probably wise to cut back if you have an excessive intake, and to limit the amount of carbonated drinks your children consume. Instead, why not offer a glass of cold milk?

NOTES TO THE COOK

To minimize the fat content of the dishes, all milk should be partially skimmed, unless specifed in the ingredients. Also, because a high sodium intake is not good for your bones, or your general health, the sodium content of the recipes has been kept as low as possible. If you do add salt, keep it to a minimum.

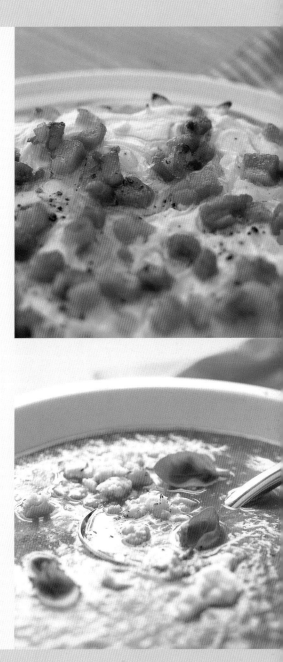

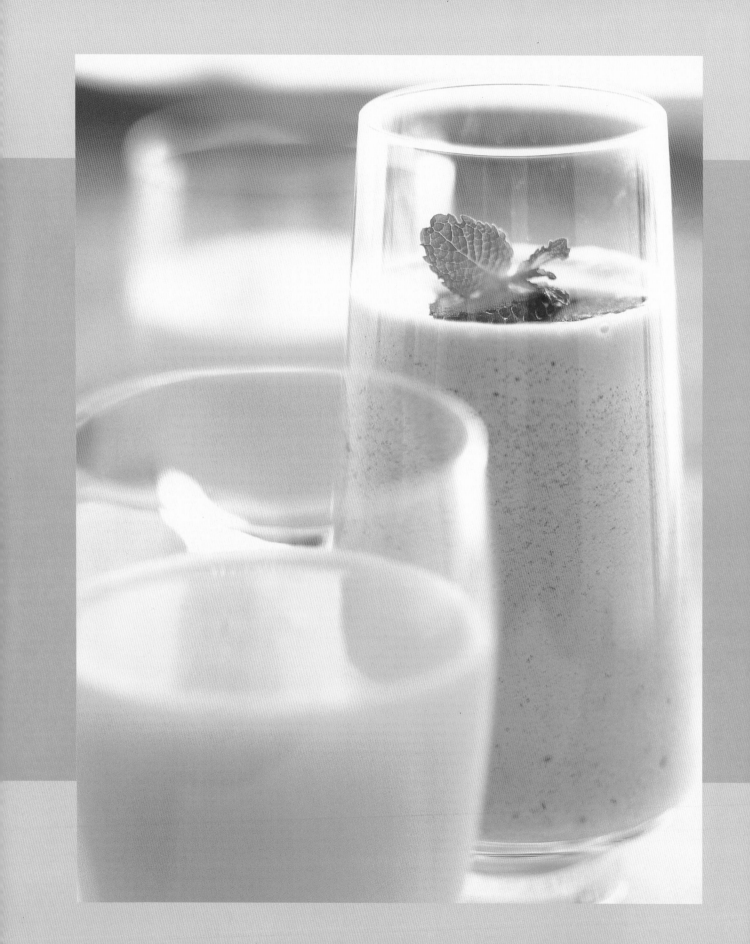

1

Start the Day

WHETHER YOU PREFER A SWEET OR SAVORY BREAKFAST, THIS CHAPTER OFFERS A VARIETY OF CALCIUM-RICH RECIPES THAT WILL GIVE YOU THE BEST POSSIBLE START TO THE DAY.

SWEET FRUIT OATMEAL

*Extra sweetness is released from the dried fruit when it is puréed,
so you don't need to add any sugar or honey.*

1 cup (250 ml) raisins or
chopped dried dates

⅔ cup (150 ml) water

⅔ cup (150 ml) milk

3 cups (750 ml) rolled oats

Pinch of salt

Serves 4

1 In a blender or food processor, blend the raisins or chopped dates with the water and milk until smooth.

2 In a heavy-based saucepan, combine the fruit mixture with the oats and add a pinch of salt. Bring to a boil, stirring steadily. Simmer the mixture, uncovered, stirring occasionally, for 4–5 minutes until the desired consistency is reached. Serve with extra milk, if desired.

APPLE & BLUEBERRY GRANOLA

Soaking the oats in apple juice gives this a delicious fruity flavor.

5 tablespoons (75 ml) rolled oats

2 tablespoons (30 ml) raisins

2 tablespoons (30 ml) slivered almonds

½ cup (125 ml) apple juice

1 cup (250 ml) plain yogurt

1 cup (250 ml) 2% milk

1 tablespoon (15 ml) clear honey

2 crisp eating apples, cored and grated

½ cup (125 ml) fresh blueberries

Serves 2–3

1 Mix together the oats, raisins, almonds, and apple juice and allow to stand for a few minutes, until the juice is absorbed.

2 Stir the yogurt, milk, honey, and grated apple into the oats and leave to stand for 15 minutes.

3 Stir in the blueberries and serve.

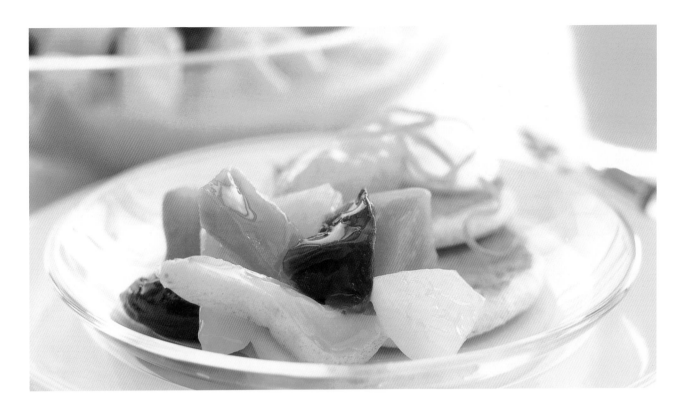

SPICED FRUIT COMPOTE

Dried fruits are useful source of calcium, particularly for people on dairy-free diets. They also make a tasty snack in between meals. This compote can also be served with natural yogurt as a dessert.

1 Put the dried fruit, cinnamon stick, and crushed cardamom in a large bowl. Add the apple and mango juice and 1¾ cups (450 ml) of boiling water. Allow to cool, cover, and leave overnight in the fridge.

2 Remove the cardamom and cinnamon stick. Mix the cornstarch with enough cold water to make a smooth paste. Drain the liquid from the fruit and place in a small saucepan. Stir in the cornstarch paste and bring to a boil. Cook for 1 minute, or until thickened, then pour over the compote. Set aside and leave to cool.

3 Place 2 pancakes on each of 4 plates with a large spoonful of the fruit compote and top with a large spoonful of yogurt. Sprinkle with orange zest to serve.

Note: To make strained yogurt, leave yogurt to set in a sieve lined with a coffee filter or paper towel for 60 minutes, longer if desired. Discard liquid.

½ lb (250 g) mixed dried fruit, such as apricots, apples and prunes or papaya, mango and pineapple

1 stick cinnamon

3 green cardamom pods, lightly crushed

1 cup (250 ml) apple juice

1 cup (250 ml) mango juice

2 teaspoons (10 ml) cornstarch

TO SERVE

8 pancakes

4 tablespoons (60 ml) strained yogurt

Zest of 1 orange

Serves 4

DRIED FRUIT SPREAD

1½ cups (325 ml) dried apricots, roughly chopped

1½ cups (325 ml) dried figs, roughly chopped

½ cup (125 ml) dried apple, roughly chopped

Zest of 1 orange

1 cup (250 ml) unsweetened orange juice

Makes 1 lb (450 g)

This is a healthier alternative to jelly or marmalade and is delicious spread on warm, buttered toast or bread. You could also try stirring a tablespoon of the spread into low-fat plain yogurt. It will keep for 3 weeks if stored in jars in the fridge.

1   Place the apricots, figs, apple, orange zest, and juice into a pan and bring to a boil. Reduce the heat and simmer for 20–30 minutes, or until the mixture is thick and the orange juice has evaporated. You can add a little more orange juice if necessary, but the final purée should be quite thick.

2   Transfer the mixture to a blender and purée until smooth. Spoon the spread into jars and store in the fridge.

BAGELS WITH RASPBERRIES & RICOTTA

¼ lb (100 g) fresh raspberries

¾ cup (175 ml) ricotta cheese

1 tablespoon (15 ml) confectioners' sugar

2 cinnamon or fruit bagels, halved

Serves 2

Ricotta cheese contains a lot less fat than most other creamy cheeses, but still provides useful amounts of calcium.

1   Place the raspberries, ricotta, and sugar in a bowl and mash until combined. Place in the fridge until needed.

2   Lightly toast the bagels and spread with the raspberry and ricotta mixture.

BANANA & ALMOND SMOOTHIE

2 ripe bananas

2 cups (500 ml) 2% milk

⅓ cup (75 ml) ground almonds

1–2 teaspoons (5–10 ml) honey, to sweeten (optional)

Serves 2

The combination of milk and fruit in smoothies is great for strong bones. Almonds are an excellent source of vitamin E, along with the minerals calcium, magnesium, phosphorus, and copper. They also give this smoothie a rich, creamy taste.

1   Peel and slice the bananas, place in a freezer container, and freeze for at least 2 hours, or overnight.

2   Place the bananas, milk, almonds, and honey in a blender or food processor and blend until thick and frothy. Pour into glasses and serve immediately.

APRICOT & ORANGE SMOOTHIE

Both dried apricots and orange juice are useful sources of calcium, making this a good alternative to milk-based smoothies for people on dairy-free diets.

1   Place the apricots in a small saucepan and cover with 1¼ cups (300 ml) water. Bring to a boil and simmer over a low heat for 10 minutes, or until the apricots are soft.

2   Place the apricots and any remaining water in a blender. Pour in the orange juice and purée until smooth.

3   To serve, pour into glasses and add a couple of ice cubes.

1 cup (250 ml) dried apricots, chopped into small pieces

1⅔ cups (400 ml) orange juice

Serves 2

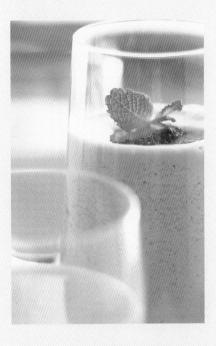

STRAWBERRY SMOOTHIE

Strawberries are rich in vitamin C, which is needed for healthy bones. The fortified soya milk is a good nondairy alternative to cow's milk and also adds vital calcium.

1   Roughly chop the strawberries and place in a plastic freezer container. Freeze for at least 2 hours, or preferably overnight.

2   Remove the strawberry pieces from the freezer. Reserve about a quarter of the strawberry pieces to decorate, then purée the remainder in a food processor or blender with the soya milk until smooth.

3   Pour the smoothie into 4 large glasses and decorate with the remaining strawberries. Garnish with mint sprigs to serve.

1 quart (1 liter) fresh ripe strawberries

2½ cups (600 ml) sweetened calcium-fortified soya milk

Fresh mint sprigs, to garnish

Serves 4

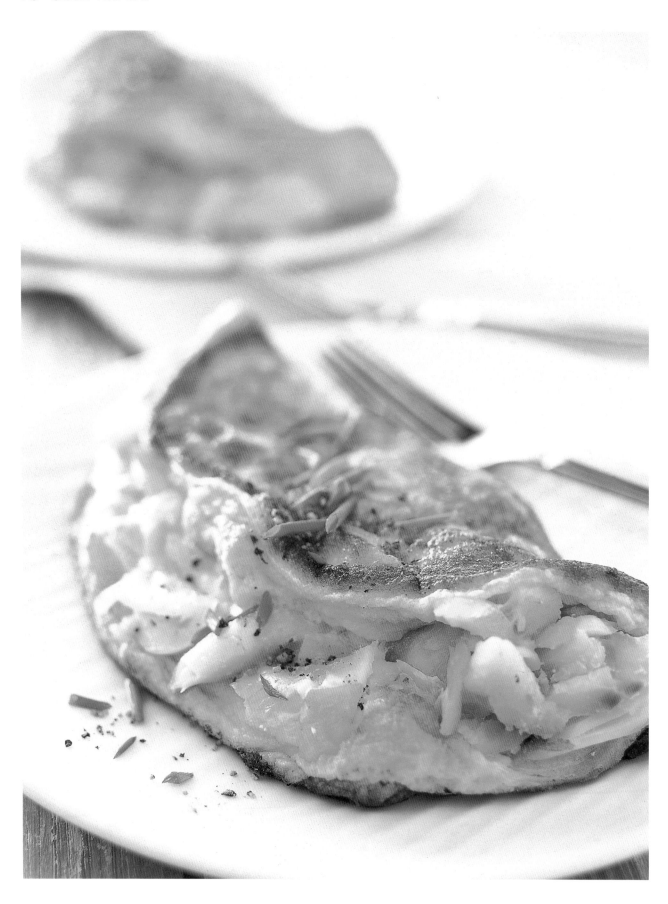

CHEESY SCRAMBLED EGGS

This breakfast provides a perfect combination of ingredients for strong bones—cheese is rich in calcium while the eggs provide vitamin D, which is essential for optimum calcium absorption.

1 Mix the eggs and milk together and season to taste. Heat the butter in a nonstick saucepan. Add the eggs and cook over a low heat, stirring continuously.

2 Once the eggs are scrambled, remove from the heat and stir in the cheese and green onions. Serve immediately on toasted whole-wheat bread.

4 eggs, beaten

2 tablespoons (30 ml) 2% milk

Salt and pepper, to taste

1 teaspoon (5 ml) butter

½ cup (125 ml) Cheddar cheese, grated

4 green onions, finely chopped

Toasted whole-wheat bread, to serve

Serves 2

SMOKED HADDOCK OMELET

This omelet is a substantial, nutritious breakfast that is quick and easy to make.

1 Place the fish in a shallow pan and cover with water. Bring to a boil, reduce the heat, and simmer gently for 5 minutes, or until the fish is cooked. Drain, then flake the fish, discarding the skin and bones.

2 Preheat the broiler. Beat the egg yolks in a bowl with the milk and seasoning. Stir in the flaked fish. Beat the egg whites until stiff then, using a metal spoon, fold into the yolk mixture.

3 Heat the butter in an omelet pan. Pour in the egg mixture and cook for 2–3 minutes or until the bottom of the omelet is set. Slide the omelet onto a flameproof serving dish.

4 Sprinkle with the cheese and place under the broiler for 2–3 minutes, or until the top has set and the cheese melted. Garnish with chives to serve.

¼ lb (125 g) smoked haddock

4 eggs, separated

2 tablespoons (30 ml) whole milk

Salt and pepper, to taste

1 tablespoon (15 ml) butter

½ cup (125 ml) Gruyère cheese, grated

Fresh chives, chopped, to garnish

Serves 2

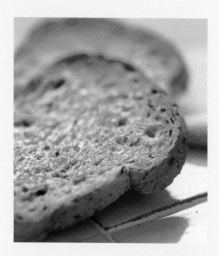

BOILED EGGS WITH SOUR CREAM & SMOKED SALMON

This is a special treat for breakfast or brunch, or a tasty and nutritious snack at any time. Both eggs and smoked salmon provide useful amounts of vitamin D, which helps the absorption of calcium. However, if you are serving this dish to anyone elderly, a pregnant woman, young children, or people who have immune deficiency disease, boil the eggs for slightly longer to make sure that they are well cooked. This will eliminate any risk of salmonella.

4 eggs

4 oz (100 g) smoked salmon

1 cup (250 ml) sour cream

1 teaspoon (5 ml) black peppercorns

Watercress, to garnish

4 slices toasted whole-grain bread, buttered, to serve

Serves 4

1　Lower the eggs into a pan of simmering water, making sure that the water covers them completely. Cook for 3½–5 minutes until soft- or hard-boiled, as preferred. Drain and rinse under cool running water, until the eggs are cool enough to handle, then shell.

2　Meanwhile, chop roughly the smoked salmon and stir into the sour cream. Crack the black peppercorns, using a pestle and mortar. If you don't have a pestle and mortar, grind the peppercorns as coarsely as you can.

3　Cut the eggs in half and arrange on individual serving plates. Spoon the smoked salmon and sour cream mixture over them. Sprinkle with the cracked black peppercorns and garnish with the cress. Serve with buttered toasted whole-grain bread.

SMOKED HADDOCK & CORN FRITTERS

Serve these light and tasty fritters with broiled tomatoes for a balanced and nutritious start to the day.

1 Place the haddock in a shallow pan and cover with the milk. Bring to a boil, then cover and simmer for 6–7 minutes, or until the fish is cooked. Remove the fish from the milk, discard the skin and bones, and flake the fish. Strain the milk and reserve.

2 Place the flour in a large bowl and make a well in the center. Whisk in the egg yolk and enough of the reserved milk to make a thick batter—you should need about ½ cup (125 ml). Stir in the corn and haddock and season to taste. In a clean bowl, beat the egg white until it forms soft peaks, then carefully fold into the batter.

3 Cook the mixture in batches by dropping spoonfuls onto a lightly greased griddle or heavy-based frying pan. Cook for 2–3 minutes, then turn carefully and cook for a further 2–3 minutes, until golden brown. Serve with the broiled tomatoes.

½ lb (200 g) smoked haddock

¾ cup (175 ml) 2% milk

¾ cup (175 ml) all-purpose flour

I egg, separated

¾ cup (175 ml) canned corn, drained

Salt and pepper, to taste

Vegetable oil, for frying

6 broiled tomatoes, halved, to serve

Serves 4 (makes 8 fritters)

STUFFED MUSHROOMS

Mushrooms are often part of breakfast dishes, and this recipe uses them in a creative and interesting way. This is a tasty and satisfying breakfast or brunch that takes just a few minutes to prepare. Serve with buttered whole-grain toasted bread.

1 Preheat the oven to 425°F (220°C). Wipe the mushrooms with a damp cloth, then remove and finely chop the stems. Lightly brush the cap of each mushroom with a little olive oil and place on a baking pan.

2 Heat the remaining oil in a large nonstick frying pan and add the chopped mushroom stems, onions, and celery. Cook over a medium heat, stirring occasionally, for 3–4 minutes, or until the vegetables are beginning to soften.

3 Stir in the bread crumbs, ham, parsley, and lemon zest, then season with salt and pepper.

4 Spoon the bread crumb mixture into the mushrooms then sprinkle with the Parmesan cheese. Bake in the oven for 15–20 minutes, or until the mushrooms are tender and golden. Garnish with sprigs of flat-leaf parsley.

8 large-capped mushrooms

2 tablespoons (30 ml) olive oil

I medium red onion, finely chopped

6 stalks celery, finely chopped

3 cups (750 ml) fine white bread crumbs

8 oz (225 g) smoked ham, very thinly sliced and roughly chopped

6 tablespoons (90 ml) fresh flat-leaf parsley, chopped

Zest of I large lemon

Salt and pepper, to taste

3 tablespoons (45 ml) Parmesan cheese, freshly grated

Sprigs of flat-leaf parsley, to garnish

Serves 4

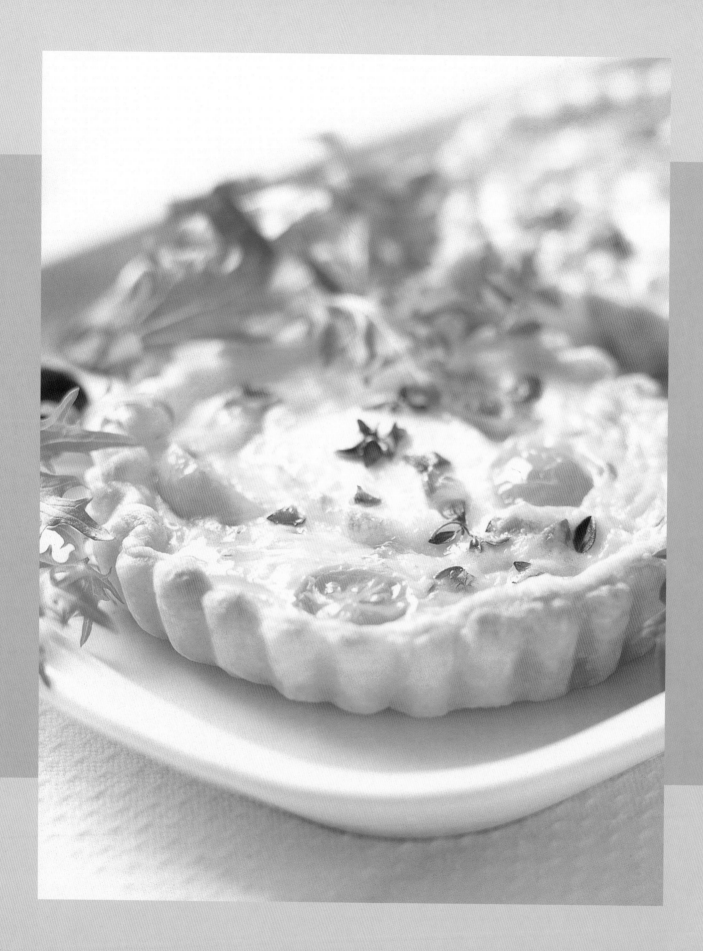

2 Soups & Appetizers

The soups and appetizers in this chapter make the most of both dairy and nondairy sources of calcium and other vitamins and minerals. Many of the recipes can be prepared in advance and served when required.

Broccoli & Stilton Soup

1 tablespoon (15 ml) vegetable oil

1 medium onion, finely chopped

1 clove garlic, peeled and finely chopped

1 large white potato, peeled and finely diced

2½ cups (600 ml) vegetable stock

1 lb (450 g) broccoli, trimmed and roughly chopped

1¼ cups (300 ml) 2% milk

Salt and pepper, to taste

1⅓ cups (325 ml) Stilton or blue cheese, crumbled

Serves 4–6

Broccoli is an excellent source of calcium and vitamin C, so is ideal as part of a bone-friendly diet. Serve this soup with crusty bread.

1 Heat the oil in large pan, then add the onion and garlic and cook for 3–4 minutes. Add the potato and continue to cook, stirring occasionally, for 2–3 minutes.

2 Add the stock and bring to a boil, then reduce the heat, cover, and cook for 10 minutes. Add the broccoli and simmer for 5–10 minutes, or until the broccoli is just tender.

3 Place the mixture in a blender and purée until smooth, then return to the pan. Stir in the milk, season to taste, and gently reheat. When the soup is hot, stir in the Stilton and, once the cheese has melted into the soup, serve.

Moroccan Spiced Chickpea Soup

2 tablespoons (30 ml) olive oil

1 large onion, chopped

1 clove garlic, peeled and finely chopped

2 medium carrots, thickly sliced

2 stalks celery, thickly sliced

2 medium zucchini, thickly sliced

2 teaspoons (10 ml) ground cumin

1 teaspoon (5 ml) turmeric

1 tablespoon (15 ml) tomato paste

14 oz (400 g) can chopped tomatoes

14 oz (400 g) can chickpeas, drained

2½ cups (600 ml) vegetable stock

3 tablespoons (45 ml) cilantro, chopped, to garnish

Serves 4

This wholesome soup is the perfect way to keep warm on a cold day. Chickpeas, along with other beans and legumes, are a useful source of calcium, particularly for people who don't eat dairy products.

1 Heat the oil in a large nonstick pan and cook the onion and garlic for 5 minutes until soft.

2 Add the carrots, celery, and zucchini and cook for a further 4–5 minutes, stirring occasionally.

3 Add the cumin and turmeric and stir to coat the vegetables. Add the tomato paste, canned tomatoes, chickpeas, and stock. Bring to a boil then cover and simmer for 20–30 minutes, until the vegetables are soft. Garnish with cilantro and serve.

ROASTED RED PEPPER SOUP WITH FETA & BASIL

The roasted red peppers give this soup a subtle sweet flavor that is enhanced by the feta and basil. To save time, you could substitute cans or jars of roasted peppers or sweet pimentos.

1 Preheat the oven to 400°F (200°C). Put the red pepper halves cut-side down on a large baking sheet and roast for 25–30 minutes or until the skins are blackened. Leave to cool slightly then put the peppers into a plastic bag for 10 minutes, until the skins loosen. Remove the skins, chop the flesh roughly, and set aside.

2 Heat the oil in a large saucepan and cook the onion and garlic for 5 minutes, until soft. Add the chopped peppers, tomatoes, vegetable stock and seasoning. Bring to a boil, cover, and simmer for 20 minutes. Remove from the heat and purée the soup in a blender or processor (you will probably need to do this in batches). Return to the pan, add the shredded basil, and reheat.

3 To serve, spoon into soup bowls and sprinkle with the feta. Garnish with basil leaves and a grinding of black pepper.

4 large red peppers, halved, cored, and seeded or 1 lb (450 g) jar roasted red peppers, drained and rinsed

2 tablespoons (30 ml) olive oil

1 large red onion, roughly chopped

2 cloves garlic, peeled and roughly chopped

14 oz (400 g) can chopped tomatoes

4 cups (1 liter) vegetable stock

Salt and pepper, to taste

2 tablespoons (30 ml) fresh basil, shredded

1 cup (250 ml) feta cheese, crumbled

Fresh basil leaves, to garnish

Serves 6

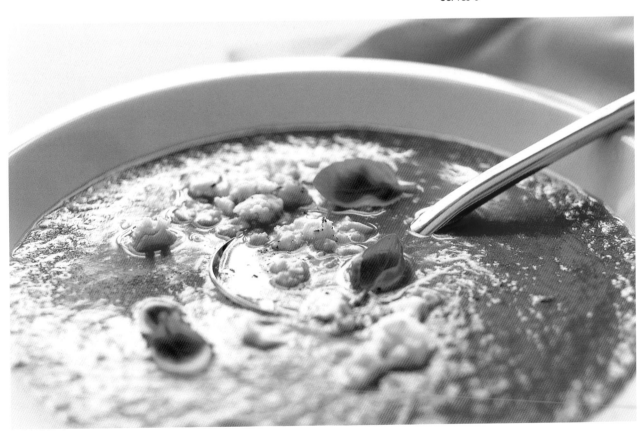

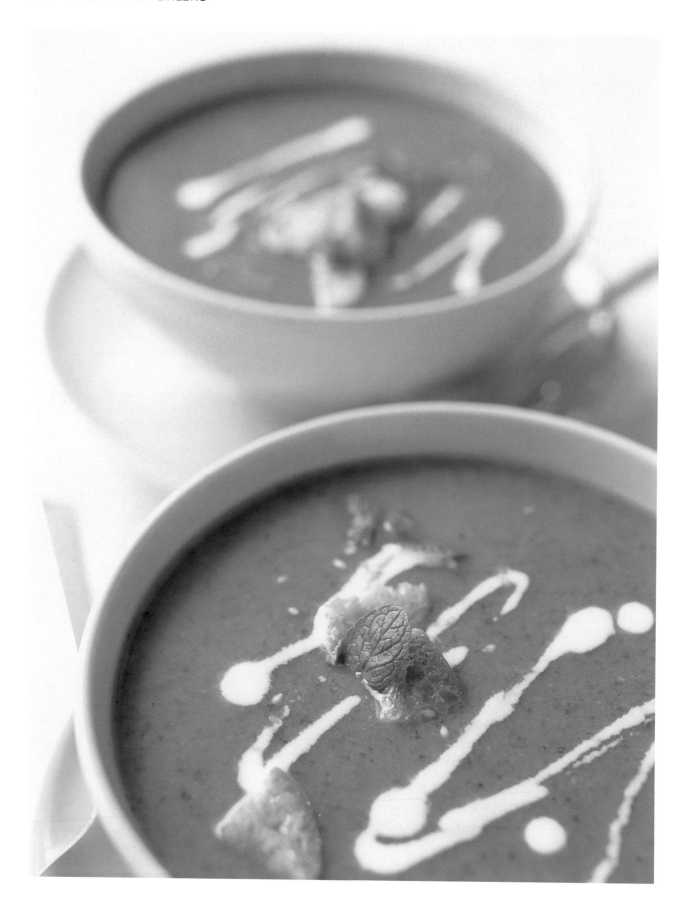

FRENCH ONION SOUP

Here, this traditional soup is served ladled over toasted bread with a sprinkling of Gruyère cheese. For a change, the Gruyère can be replaced with goat cheese, Emmenthal, mozzarella, or any blue cheese.

1 Melt the butter in a large saucepan, add the onions, and cook gently for 15–20 minutes until they are golden brown.

2 Sift the flour into the pan and cook, stirring continuously, for 1 minute. Stir in the stock, seasoning, and add the bay leaf. Bring to a boil, cover, and simmer for 30 minutes.

3 Cut the French loaf diagonally into ½ in (1 cm) slices. Heat the broiler to medium and toast the bread lightly on both sides. Place two slices in each of 4 ovenproof soup bowls and ladle the soup over them, discarding the bay leaf.

4 Turn the broiler to high. Sprinkle the Gruyère cheese over the soup and place under the broiler until the cheese is bubbling. Serve immediately.

¼ cup (50 ml) butter

3 large onions, thinly sliced

1 tablespoon (15 ml) all-purpose flour

4 cups (1 liter) vegetable stock

Salt and pepper, to taste

1 bay leaf

½ medium French loaf

¾ cup (175 ml) Gruyère cheese, grated

Serves 4

GARDEN PEA & WATERCRESS SOUP WITH SESAME CROÛTONS

The bright color of this creamy, fresh-tasting soup makes it an eye-catching appetizer, while the sesame croûtons add texture and interest.

1 To make the croûtons, brush the bread pieces with 2 tablespoons (30 ml) of the oil and sprinkle with the sesame seeds. Heat the remaining oil in a nonstick pan and cook the croûtons over a high heat for 3–4 minutes until crisp and golden. Remove and drain on paper towel, then set aside to cool.

2 To make the soup, melt the butter in a large saucepan. Add the onion and cook for 5 minutes until soft, then add the peas, watercress, stock, and seasoning. Bring slowly to a boil, lower the heat, cover, and simmer for 5 minutes.

3 Allow the soup to cool slightly, then process in a blender or food processor until smooth (you will probably need to do this in batches). Pour into a clean saucepan, season to taste, and reheat.

4 Drizzle with crème fraîche or heavy cream and garnish with chopped mint and the sesame croûtons. Serve with chunks of whole-wheat or whole-grain bread.

FOR THE SESAME CROÛTONS

3 slices ciabatta or French bread, cut into small pieces

3 tablespoons (45 ml) olive oil

1 tablespoon (15 ml) sesame seeds

FOR THE SOUP

2½ tablespoons (40 ml) butter

1 large onion, finely chopped

1 lb (450 g) fresh or frozen peas

¾ cup (175 ml) fresh watercress, chopped

4 cups (1 liter) hot vegetable stock

Salt and pepper, to taste

4–6 tablespoons (60–90 ml) crème fraîche or heavy cream, to garnish

Fresh mint leaves, to garnish

Serves 4–6

SMOKED HADDOCK & CORN CHOWDER

2 tablespoons (30 ml) butter

I medium onion, peeled and finely chopped

2 medium white potatoes, peeled and cut into small cubes

1⅔ cups (400 ml) fish stock

10½ oz (300 g) can corn, drained

1⅔ cups (400 ml) 2% milk

I lb (450 g) skinless smoked haddock fillets, cut into bite-sized pieces

Salt and pepper, to taste

Fresh parsley, chopped, to garnish

Serves 4

Using 2% milk gives this soup a creamy rich taste, while reducing the fat content of the dish. It is also a good source of calcium. The soup is delicious served with crusty bread.

1 Melt the butter in a large saucepan, add the onion, and cook over a gentle heat for 5 minutes until soft. Add the potato and continue cooking for a further 2 minutes.

2 Add the fish stock and bring to a boil. Reduce the heat, cover and simmer for about 10–15 minutes, or until the potatoes are tender. Roughly mash the potatoes.

3 Add the corn and milk and return to a boil. Reduce the heat and simmer for 5 minutes. Stir in the fish and continue to cook for a further 5 minutes. Season to taste and garnish with chopped parsley.

BAKED RICOTTA WITH ROASTED VINE TOMATOES

Butter, for greasing dish

3 cups (750 ml) ricotta cheese

1¼ cups (300 ml) Parmesan cheese, freshly grated

2 eggs, separated

Salt and pepper, to taste

4 plum tomatoes, halved

I tablespoon (15 ml) olive oil

I tablespoon (15 ml) balsamic vinegar

Serves 4

This dish is ideal as an appetizer or a light lunch with a green salad. Mixing Parmesan cheese with the ricotta cheese boosts the flavor as well as the calcium content.

1 Preheat the oven to 350°F (180°C). Grease a shallow ovenproof dish.

2 Place the ricotta and the Parmesan cheeses in a bowl and beat in the egg yolks until the mixture is smooth. Season to taste.

3 In a clean bowl, beat the egg whites until stiff. Using a metal spoon, fold the egg whites into the cheese mixture.

4 Spoon the mixture into the prepared dish and bake for 30–40 minutes, or until slightly risen, golden, and firm to the touch. Allow to cool.

5 Place the tomatoes cut-side up on a baking tray. Mix the olive oil and balsamic vinegar together and drizzle over the tomatoes. Season and bake for 20 minutes, or until the tomatoes are softened and slightly charred.

6 Slice the baked cheese into quarters and serve with the tomatoes.

MUSHROOMS & GOAT CHEESE IN EGGPLANT PARCELS

These tasty parcels are ideal as an appetizer, and an arugula or spring mix salad with balsamic dressing makes a good accompaniment. Mushrooms are rich in copper, which is a vital mineral for strong bones.

1   Cut the eggplant lengthwise into thin slices. Sprinkle with salt and set aside for 30 minutes. Rinse well and pat dry with paper towel. Brush the eggplant with 1 tablespoon (15 ml) oil and place under a hot broiler for 2–3 minutes on each side, until golden brown. Transfer to a plate lined with paper towel and set aside.

2   Heat the remaining oil in large nonstick frying pan, add the garlic, green onions, and mushrooms and cook for 10–15 minutes, until all the liquid has evaporated. Set aside to cool.

3   Combine the mushroom mixture and the goat cheese and season to taste. Line the base and sides of two 6-oz (150-ml) ramekin dishes with the broiled eggplant slices, allowing about one third of the slices to hang over the edge. Spoon the mushroom and cheese mixture into the ramekins and fold over the eggplant slices to encase the mixture. Chill for 15 minutes.

4   Preheat oven to 375°F (190°C). Turn the parcels out onto a lightly oiled baking sheet and bake in oven for 10–15 minutes until cooked. Serve immediately.

1 long, thin eggplant
Salt, for sprinkling eggplant
2 tablespoons (30 ml) olive oil
1 clove garlic, peeled and finely chopped
4 green onions, finely chopped
1¼ cups (300 ml) button mushrooms, finely chopped
4 oz (125 g) soft goat cheese, rind removed
Salt and pepper, to taste
Serves 2

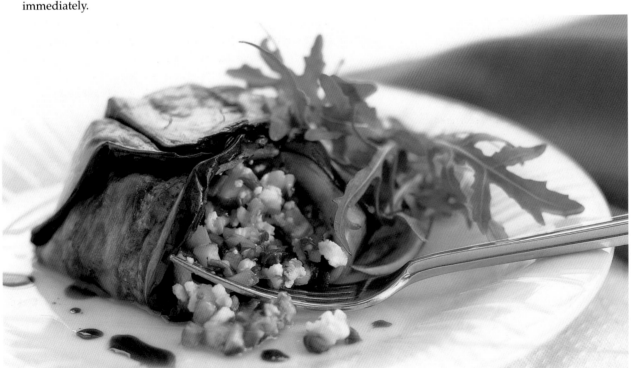

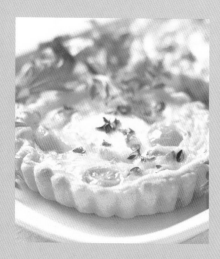

CHERRY TOMATO & GOAT CHEESE TARTLETS

These crisp individual pastries have a rich cheese and tomato filling and make a great appetizer. They also make a delicious lunchtime snack, accompanied by a leafy green salad.

1 Preheat the oven to 400°F (200°C). On a lightly floured surface, roll out the puff pastry and use to line four 4-in (10-cm) tartlet pans. Line the pastry cases with baking parchment and fill with baking beans. Chill for 10 minutes.

2 Bake the pastry cases for 10 minutes. Remove the paper and beans and bake for a further 10 minutes, until the pastry is lightly golden.

3 Meanwhile, heat the oil in a nonstick frying pan. Add the red onion and thyme. Cook gently for 3–4 minutes until soft. Remove from the heat and set aside.

4 Beat the eggs and cream together. Add the Gruyère cheese and cooled onion mixture. Season and mix well. Cut the goat cheese into 4 round slices. Divide the egg mixture into the tartlets and put 4 cherry tomato halves and 1 goat cheese slice in each tartlet.

5 Bake the tartlets for 15 minutes until the filling is set. Cool slightly before removing them from the tins. Scatter a few thyme leaves over the warm tartlets just before serving.

Flour, for dusting

½ lb (225 g) ready-made puff pastry

1 tablespoon (15 ml) olive oil

1 medium red onion, finely chopped

1 teaspoon (5 ml) fresh thyme, chopped

2 eggs

⅔ cup (150 ml) light cream

¼ cup (50 ml) Gruyère cheese, finely grated

Salt and pepper, to taste

4 oz (125 g) firm, round goat cheese

8 cherry tomatoes, halved

Few fresh thyme leaves, to garnish

Serves 4

TOMATO & MOZZARELLA SALAD

A classic combination that makes a tasty appetizer or a welcome accompaniment to most Italian dishes. If you're watching your fat intake, choose low-fat mozzarella cheese; although it contains less fat, it is still a good source of calcium. Serve with crusty bread.

1 Whisk together the oil and vinegar to make the dressing. Season to taste.

2 Arrange the tomatoes and mozzarella cheese on a large plate. Drizzle with the dressing and sprinkle the basil over the top.

6 tablespoons (90 ml) olive oil

2 tablespoons (30 ml) white wine vinegar

Salt and pepper, to taste

3 large beefsteak tomatoes, thickly sliced

2 6-oz (150-g) round mozzarella cheeses, thickly sliced

Handful fresh basil, roughly torn

Serves 4–6

WATERCRESS, PEAR & ROQUEFORT SALAD

The contrasting flavors in this salad make it an interesting snack, appetizer, or accompaniment. Roquefort, watercress, and almonds are all rich in bone-strengthening calcium. Serve with crusty bread.

1 To make the dressing, whisk together the oil, vinegar, mustard, and salt.

2 Place the watercress in a large serving bowl. Peel, core, and slice the pears and mix into the watercress, along with the cheese and almonds. Drizzle over the dressing and toss.

FOR THE DRESSING

5 tablespoons (60 ml) olive oil

1 tablespoon (15 ml) white wine vinegar

½ teaspoon (2 ml) mustard powder

Pinch of salt

FOR THE SALAD

1½ cups (375 ml) watercress, washed

2 ripe pears

2 cups (500 ml) Roquefort cheese, crumbled

½ cup (125 ml) slivered almonds, toasted

Serves 4

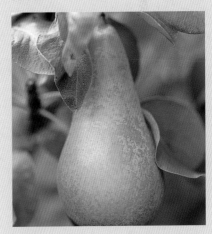

AVOCADO & SMOKED SALMON ROLLS

Low-fat soft cheese contains considerably less fat than full-fat cheese, but still contains good amounts of calcium. Oil-rich fish, such as salmon, provide vitamin D, which is essential for the absorption of calcium. These rolls are delicious served with whole-wheat toast.

1 Remove the flesh of the avocado and mash. Add the cheese, lemon juice and seasoning and mix well. Chill the mixture in the fridge for 15 minutes.

2 Place the strips of salmon on a sheet of waxed paper or plastic wrap and spread with the avocado mixture. Roll the salmon, from the shortest side, to enclose the avocado. Wrap the salmon rolls in waxed paper or plastic wrap and place in the fridge until needed—they can prepared up to 4 hours in advance. To serve, remove wrap and garnish with lemon wedges.

1 medium-ripe avocado

4 oz (125 g) low-fat soft cheese

Juice of half a lemon

Salt and pepper, to taste

4 oz (125 g) smoked salmon, cut into 4 strips, each about 4 × 3 in (12 × 9 cm)

Lemon wedges, to garnish

Serves 2

ROASTED RED PEPPER DIP

2 large red peppers, halved

4 oz (125 g) low-fat cream cheese

2 teaspoons (10 ml) sweet chili sauce

Salt and pepper, to taste

Serves 2–3

This delicious red pepper dip is ideal for serving with crudités, but for a tasty, nutritious lunchtime snack, it can be spread on whole-wheat bread and topped with a few salad leaves or alfalfa sprouts.

1 Preheat the oven to 400°F (200°C). Put the pepper halves cut-side down on a large baking sheet and roast for 25–30 minutes, or until the skins are blackened. Leave to cool slightly then put into a plastic bag for 10 minutes, until the skins loosen. Peel away the skin, chop the flesh roughly, and set aside.

2 Place the peppers, cheese, chili sauce, and seasoning into a food processor or blender and process for 1–2 minutes, until smooth.

3 Cover and place in the fridge for at least 2 hours before serving to allow the flavors to develop.

TZATZIKI

½ large cucumber

1 cup (250 ml) Balkan-style yogurt

1 clove garlic, peeled and finely chopped

Salt and pepper, to taste

Serves 2–3

Tzatziki makes a delicious lower-fat alternative to creamy dips and sauces. Serve with vegetable crudités and strips of warm pita bread.

1 Slice the cucumber in half lengthwise. Seed and dice the flesh.

2 Mix the yogurt, cucumber, garlic, and seasoning together. Cover and set aside until needed.

CREAMY GUACAMOLE

4 ripe avocados

3 plum tomatoes, skinned, seeded, and diced

Juice of 1 lime

1 clove garlic, peeled and finely chopped

6 tablespoons (90 ml) Balkan-style yogurt

1 large red chili pepper, seeded and chopped (optional)

2 tablespoons (30 ml) cilantro, chopped

Salt and pepper, to taste

Serves 6

It is essential to use ripe avocados when making guacamole—they should "give" slightly when pressed at the pointed end. A hard, underripe fruit will ripen in 1–2 days at room temperature, if stored in a bowl with ripe fruit. Serve with tortilla chips and raw sliced vegetables.

1 Cut the avocados in half and remove the pits. Using a spoon, scoop the flesh into a bowl and mash thoroughly.

2 Add the tomatoes, lime juice, garlic, yogurt, red chili (if using), cilantro, and seasoning. Cover the bowl with plastic wrap to prevent discoloring, making sure there are no gaps. Chill for 1–2 hours.

3 Uncover and mix lightly once more before serving.

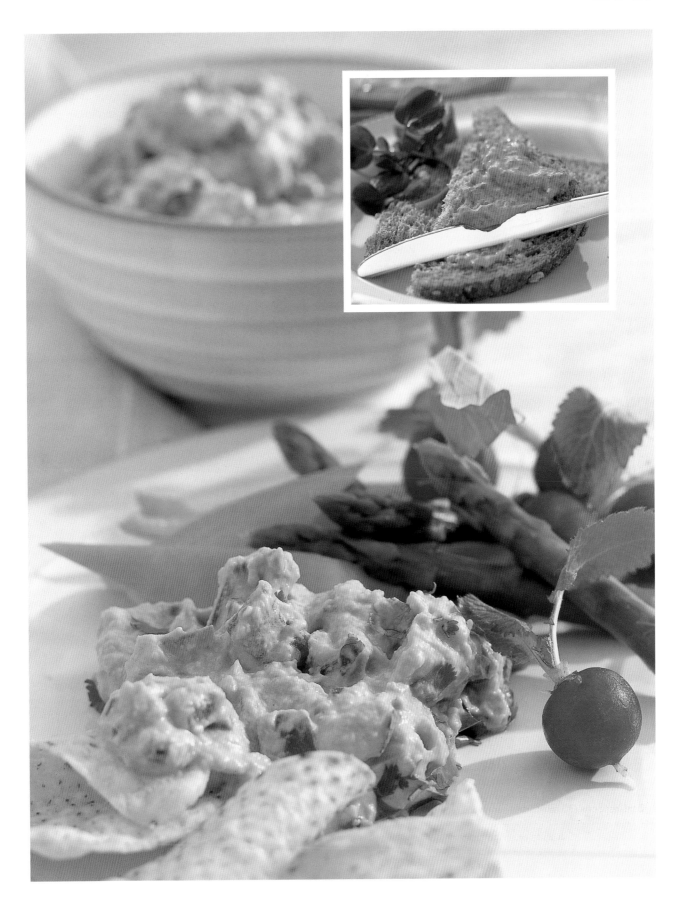

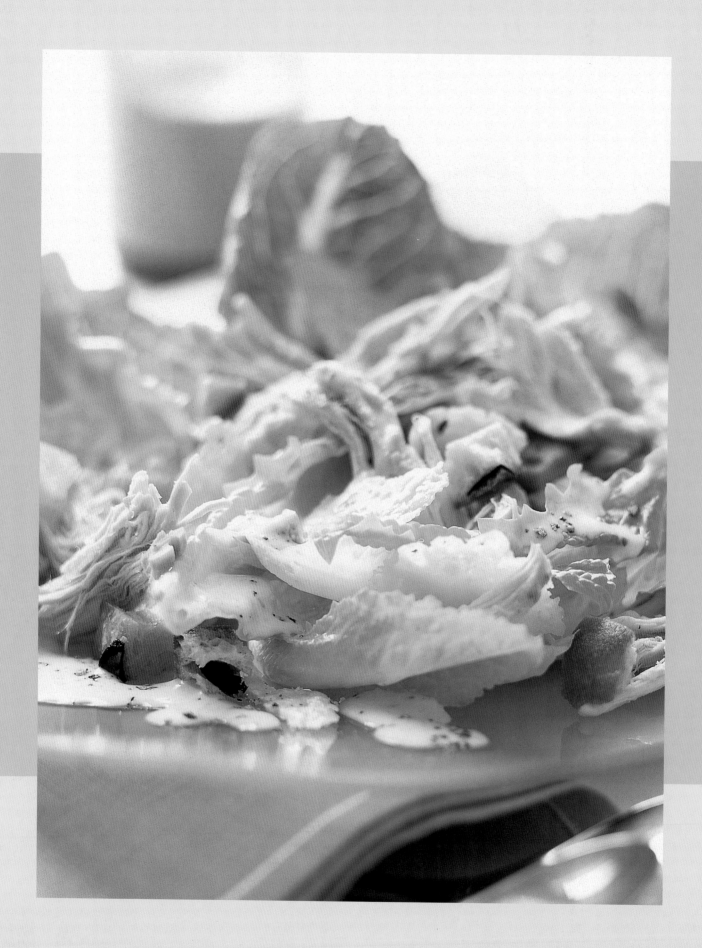

Light Snacks & Lunches

3

It's easy to resort to packaged, processed foods when we want a snack, but these often contain many unwanted additives and very few vitamins and minerals. This chapter offers quick and easy-to-prepare snacks and lunches that are both appealing and healthy.

HUMMUS

Homemade hummus is quick and easy to make and beats the store-bought variety. Cans of chickpeas are a nutritious and versatile ingredient to have on hand—apart from using them to make hummus, you can add them to salads, soups, stews, and casseroles. Tahini is a purée of sesame seeds available at stores that sell Middle Eastern food products.

14 oz (400 g) can chickpeas, drained and rinsed

2 tablespoons (30 ml) lemon juice

1 teaspoon (5 ml) ground cumin

¼ cup (50 ml) extra virgin olive oil, plus extra for drizzling

2 cloves garlic, peeled

4 tablespoons (60 ml) tahini

Cayenne pepper or paprika, for dusting

Vegetable crudités or toasted pita bread, to serve

Serves 4

1 Put the chickpeas in a food processor or blender and process until semi-smooth. Add the lemon juice, cumin, oil, garlic, and tahini and continue to blend until smooth. If the mixture is too thick, add a little more oil.

2 Place the mixture in a bowl, drizzle with a little extra virgin oil, and dust with cayenne or paprika. Serve immediately with vegetable crudités or toasted pita, or cover and chill until needed.

RED PEPPER HUMMUS

The roasted red peppers give this hummus a tangy sweet taste that is enhanced by the chili sauce. This is delicious served with vegetable crudités or spread on whole-wheat bread.

2 large red peppers

14 oz (400 g) can chickpeas, drained and rinsed

2 tablespoons (30 ml) lemon juice

1 teaspoon (5 ml) sweet chili sauce

¼ cup (50 ml) extra virgin olive oil

2 cloves garlic, peeled

3 tablespoons (45 ml) tahini

3 tablespoons (45 ml) hot water

Serves 4

1 Halve the peppers and place under a hot broiler for about 20 minutes or until the skins are black. Cover with a clean wet cloth, or place in a plastic bag, and allow to cool for about 10 minutes. Remove the skin from the peppers and blot dry with paper towel.

2 Place the peppers, chickpeas, lemon juice, sweet chili sauce, olive oil, garlic, tahini and hot water in a food processor or blender and process until smooth. Serve immediately, or cover and chill until needed.

FALAFEL WITH SALAD IN PITA

Chickpeas are a useful source of fiber, B vitamins and minerals. This recipe makes a hearty and nutritious light lunch.

1 Preheat the oven to 350°F (180°C). To make the falafel, mash the chickpeas with the onion and garlic to form a thick pulp. Add the tahini, egg, bread crumbs, cilantro, cumin, and salt and mix together well.

2 Divide the falafel mixture into 18 small balls and bake on a baking pan for 15–20 minutes, or until lightly golden and firm to the touch.

3 To serve, toast the pita breads, leave to cool slightly and split open. Fill with the shredded lettuce, cherry tomatoes, and cucumber. Top the salad with 3 falafel per pita and drizzle with a little hummus, if you like. Sprinkle with a little cayenne pepper or paprika.

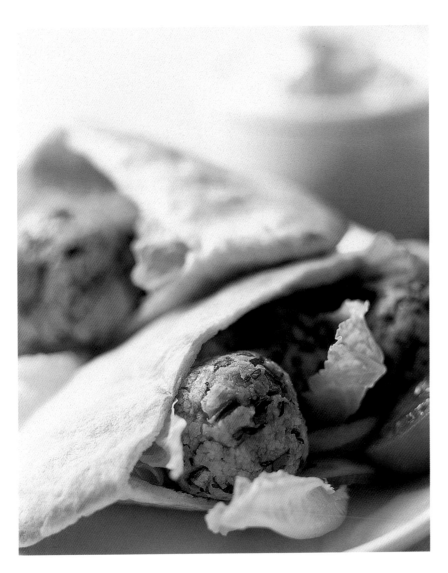

FOR THE FALAFEL

14 oz (400 g) can chickpeas, drained and rinsed

1 red onion, roughly chopped

1 clove garlic, peeled and crushed

3 tablespoons (45 ml) tahini

1 egg, beaten

2 cups (500 ml) fresh white bread crumbs

2 tablespoons (30 ml) cilantro, chopped

1 teaspoon (5 ml) ground cumin

½ teaspoon (2 ml) salt

TO SERVE

6 large pita breads

Shredded romaine lettuce leaves

Cherry tomatoes, halved

½ cucumber, sliced

Hummus (see recipe page 34)

Cayenne pepper or paprika, for sprinkling

Serves 6

QUICK CIABATTA PIZZA

A quick and healthy lunchtime snack or light supper dish, this can be served on its own or accompanied by a fresh green salad.

4 ciabatta rolls or 1 loaf French bread

3 tablespoons (45 ml) sun-dried tomato paste or red pesto

1 tablespoon (15 ml) fresh basil leaves, chopped

3 plum tomatoes, thinly sliced

10 oz (285 g) jar artichoke hearts in oil, drained and roughly chopped

4 oz (125 g) soft rindless goat cheese, crumbled

1 tablespoon (15 ml) hazelnuts, chopped

Black pepper, to taste

Olive oil, for drizzling

Fresh basil leaves, to garnish

Serves 4

1   Preheat the oven to 400°F (200°C). Cut the ciabatta rolls in half and arrange cut-side up on a baking pan.

2   Spread the sun-dried tomato paste or red pesto over the cut surface of each toasted roll. Sprinkle with the chopped basil. Place a layer of tomato slices over the pesto and basil, then top with artichoke hearts and goat cheese. Sprinkle with the hazelnuts. Season well with black pepper and drizzle with a little olive oil.

3   Bake in the oven for about 10 minutes, or until heated through. Garnish with basil leaves.

CROQUE MONSIEUR

This quick snack is great served with a simple mixed salad. If cooking for two people, double all the ingredients except the oil—if necessary, use two pans or cook in batches.

2 slices white or whole-wheat bread

1 tablespoon (15 ml) butter

1 slice good quality ham

2 oz (50 g) slice Gruyère or Swiss cheese

Salt and pepper, to taste

2 teaspoons (10 ml) vegetable oil

Serves 1

1   Cut the crusts off the bread, then spread one side of each with some of the butter. Place the ham on the buttered side of one slice of bread, cutting to fit if necessary, and cover with the Gruyère or Swiss cheese. Season and top with the remaining slice of bread, buttered side down.

2   Press the sandwich together firmly, then cut into 4 triangles.

3   Melt the remaining butter with the oil in a nonstick frying pan. Fry the triangles over a moderate heat, turning once, until golden on both sides. Press with a spatula to keep the sandwiches together. Serve hot.

WELSH RAREBIT

Place ½ cup (125 ml) grated Cheddar cheese, 1 tablespoon (15 ml) butter, 1 tablespoon (15 ml) dark beer, ½ teaspoon (2 ml) mustard, and seasoning in a saucepan. Heat very gently, stirring continuously, until the mixture becomes thick and creamy. Lightly toast one side of a slice of bread. Pour the sauce over the uncooked side and cook under a preheated hot broiler until it is golden and bubbling. Serve with a crisp green salad. For "buck rarebit," top with a poached egg.

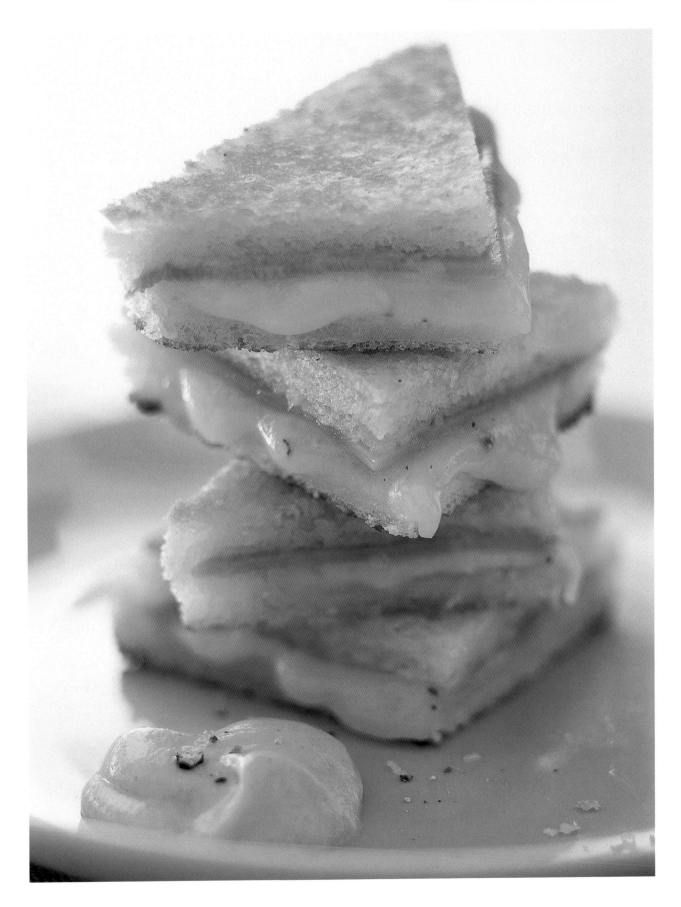

PEPPERED SMOKED MACKEREL SPREAD

10 oz (285 g) peppered smoked mackerel fillets

7 oz (200 g) cream cheese with herbs and garlic

2 tablespoons (30 ml) fresh flat-leaf parsley, chopped

Zest and juice of 1 lemon

Serves 4

A quick and easy fish spread made with cream cheese and a hint of lemon. It can be made in advance and frozen, but remember to defrost it thoroughly before serving. Serve with a green salad and toasted whole-grain bread.

1 Remove the skin from the smoked mackerel along with any small bones. Flake the fish into a bowl.

2 Add the soft cheese, flat-leaf parsley, lemon zest and juice to the fish and mash together with a fork. Spoon the mixture into a serving bowl. Cover and chill until required.

CHICKEN TIKKA SALAD

4 tablespoons (60 ml) plain yogurt

4 tablespoons (60 ml) mayonnaise

4 tablespoons (60 ml) grated cucumber

3 green onions, finely chopped

2 teaspoons (10 ml) fresh mint, chopped

Salt and pepper, to taste

Mixed salad greens

1 lb (450 g) chicken tikka

Sprigs of fresh mint, to garnish

Serves 4

Mixing the mayonnaise with plain yogurt reduces the fat and boosts the calcium content of this dish. Serve with toasted pita bread.

1 Mix the yogurt with the mayonnaise, cucumber, green onions and mint, blending well to make a dressing. Season to taste. Cover and chill until ready to use.

2 Just before serving, arrange the salad greens on a large serving plate and top with the chicken tikka. Spoon the cucumber, mint, and yogurt dressing over the chicken and garnish with sprigs of fresh mint.

Note: Chicken tikka is a popular Anglo-Indian dish based on tandoori chicken. Smoked chicken/turkey would be a good substitute.

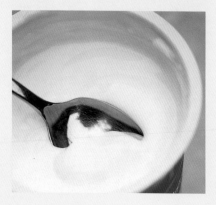

CHICKEN CAESAR SALAD WITH PARMESAN CRISPS

The Parmesan crisps in this salad provide plenty of calcium. When serving salads, it is best to put the dressing on at the last moment, as this stops the leaves going soggy.

1   To make the croûtons, cut the bread roughly into small pieces. Heat the olive oil in a large frying pan. Add the bread pieces and cook over a high heat for 3 minutes, stirring occasionally, until crisp and golden. Set aside to cool.

2   Preheat the oven to 400°F (200°C). On a large baking pan, make 8 heaped piles of grated Parmesan cheese, spacing them well apart. Bake for about 5 minutes until the cheese melts, then remove from the oven and leave to cool.

3   On a chopping board, shred the chicken into bite-sized pieces. Tear the lettuce into pieces and put into a large bowl, then toss in a little of the Caesar salad dressing.

4   Pile the lettuce onto 4 large plates, and top with the chicken. Sprinkle with the croûtons, then drizzle with the remaining Caesar dressing. Break the Parmesan crisps into pieces and sprinkle over the salad. Season with black pepper.

4 slices black olive ciabatta or French bread

2 tablespoons (30 ml) olive oil

1¼ cups (300 ml) Parmesan cheese, freshly grated

3 cooked chicken breast fillets

Inside leaves of 1 romaine lettuce

4–5 tablespoons (60–75 ml) Caesar salad dressing

Black pepper, to taste

Serves 4

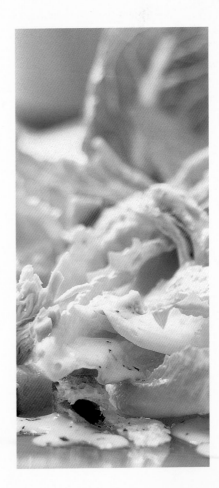

CAESAR SALAD ON TOASTED CIABATTA
Mix together 1 thinly sliced red onion, 2 shredded green onions, 4 halved cherry tomatoes, ¼ sliced cucumber, and 1 tablespoon (15 ml) extra virgin olive oil. Season well. Preheat the broiler to high. Slice a ciabatta lengthwise, then cut the 2 pieces in half and toast for 1–2 minutes. Drizzle a little olive oil onto the toasted ciabatta, then place 1 romaine lettuce leaf on each piece. Fill each leaf with shredded cooked chicken and the salad mixture. Spoon the Caesar dressing over the salad, top with Parmesan shavings, and season with black pepper.

HOME-MADE CAESAR SALAD DRESSING
Put 3 chopped cloves of garlic in a saucepan with ⅔ cup (150 ml) white wine. Bring to a boil and simmer for 5 minutes. Leave to cool, then put in a food processor or blender with ½ cup (125 ml) grated Parmesan cheese, 4 egg yolks, 1 tablespoon (15 ml) Dijon mustard, 2 anchovy fillets and 1 teaspoon (5 ml) white wine vinegar. Blend until well emulsified, then add 1¼ cups (300 ml) olive oil in a steady stream, until the dressing is smooth. Season well. Store in a jar and keep, refrigerated, for up to 1 week.

FETA OMELET WITH ARUGULA & RED PEPPER

4 large eggs, separated

2 tablespoons (30 ml) fresh mixed herbs, chopped

1⅔ cups (400 ml) feta cheese, roughly crumbled

Black pepper, to taste

1 tablespoon (15 ml) butter

1¼ cups (300 ml) red or mixed peppers in oil, drained and sliced

½ cup (125 ml) small arugula leaves

Serves 2

This light and fluffy cheese omelet makes a quick and tasty dish. Serve with a simple plum tomato salad.

1 Preheat the broiler to high. Beat the egg yolks with 3 tablespoons of water, then stir in the herbs, half the feta, and plenty of black pepper. In a clean bowl, whisk the egg whites until stiff, then fold into the egg yolk mixture.

2 Over a medium heat, melt the butter in a large nonstick frying pan until foamy, then spoon in the egg mixture. Cook for 3–4 minutes until the underside of the omelet is golden. Remove from the heat and place under the broiler for 2–3 minutes, until the top of the omelet is lightly brown.

3 Sprinkle the pepper slices and the remaining feta evenly over the top of the omelet. Return to the broiler and cook for a further 2–3 minutes until the feta begins to melt slightly. Place the arugula evenly on top of the red pepper and feta and season with black pepper.

4 Fold the omelet in half, then cut in half and serve.

TWICE-BAKED GOAT CHEESE SOUFFLÉS

2½ tablespoons (40 ml) butter, plus extra for greasing

¼ cup (50 ml) Parmesan cheese, freshly grated, plus extra for sprinkling

2 tablespoons (30 ml) pastry flour

scant 1 cup (225 ml) 2% milk

2 medium eggs, separated

4 oz (125 g) soft rindless goat cheese, crumbled

Salt and pepper, to taste

Serves 4

These light and tasty soufflés can be served with a crisp green salad and some whole-wheat bread for a healthy lunchtime snack. They also make a good appetizer at a dinner party.

1 Lightly grease four 6-oz (150-ml) ramekins and sprinkle Parmesan cheese over the base and the sides of the ramekins until evenly coated.

2 Preheat the oven to 350°F (180°C). Melt the butter in a saucepan, then stir in the flour and cook for 1 minute, stirring constantly. Gradually stir in the milk. Bring to a boil and cook for 2–3 minutes, or until the sauce becomes thick and smooth.

3 Allow the sauce to cool slightly then beat in the egg yolks, goat cheese, and seasoning. Whisk the egg whites until they form soft peaks, then, using a metal spoon, carefully fold into the cheese sauce.

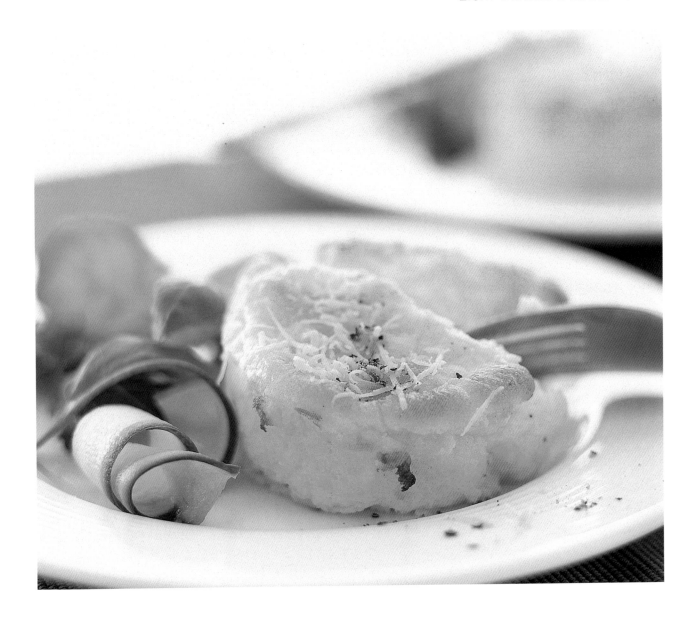

4 Divide the mixture into the ramekins and place in a roasting pan. Fill the
   pan with enough boiling water to reach halfway up the sides of the
   ramekins and place in the oven for 20–25 minutes, or until the soufflés are
   firm to the touch and lightly browned. Remove from the roasting pan and
   allow to cool. Run a knife around the edge of each soufflé and carefully
   turn out. Chill until ready to serve.

5 About 30 minutes before serving, heat the oven to 400°F (200°C). Carefully
   transfer the soufflés to a lightly greased baking pan, sprinkle with
   Parmesan cheese, and bake for 15–20 minutes or until golden brown.

BLUE CHEESE SOUFFLÉS
Replace the goat cheese with Stilton or another blue cheese.

SPINACH & ROQUEFORT CRÊPES

You can use any strong cheese to make these crêpes, but the combination of salty Roquefort and spinach works particularly well.

¾ cup (175 ml) sifted all-purpose flour

I egg, beaten

Pinch of salt

I¼ cups (300 ml) 2% milk

Vegetable oil, for frying

I lb (500 g) fresh spinach, washed

2 cups (500 ml) Roquefort or other blue cheese, chopped into small pieces

Serves 4 (makes 8 small crêpes)

1   Mix the flour, egg, and salt together in a large bowl. Gradually beat in enough milk to make a smooth batter with the consistency of light cream. Let stand for about 20 minutes.

2   Heat a small pan. When the pan is hot, brush with a little oil and pour in enough batter to thinly coat the base of the pan. Cook over a medium heat for about 1 minute, or until the edges are curling away from the pan and the underside is golden. Flip the crêpe and cook for a further 30 seconds, then turn out onto a sheet of waxed paper. Add a little more oil to the pan and repeat the process until all the batter has been used. Cover the crêpes to keep them warm.

3   Place the spinach in a large saucepan with 1 tablespoon (15 ml) of water. Cover and cook until the leaves are just wilted. Squeeze out any excess liquid, then chop roughly. Return to the pan and gently reheat.

4   Spoon a little of the spinach into the middle of each crêpe and sprinkle over a little of the cheese. Fold the crêpes in half to serve.

CAJUN CHEESE POTATO SKINS WITH TOMATO & RED ONION SALAD

These are guaranteed to be a big hit with the whole family. Served with a salad, they are ideal for a light lunch, or with grilled chicken or fish for a more substantial meal.

FOR THE POTATO SKINS

4 baking potatoes

Oil, for brushing

2 tablespoons (30 ml) Cajun seasoning mix

8 thin slices of Cheddar cheese, cut in half

1   Preheat the oven to 400°F (200°C). Push a metal skewer through each potato (this speeds up the cooking process by about 20 minutes) and bake for 1 hour or until tender.

2   Remove the potatoes from the oven and set aside to cool slightly. Turn the oven up to 425°F (225°C). Remove the skewers and carefully cut each potato into 6 wedges.

3   Brush each potato wedge with a little oil, then dust on both sides with the Cajun seasoning. Put the wedges on a baking pan and return to the oven for a further 15–20 minutes, until crispy and golden.

4   Meanwhile, make the salad. Slice the tomatoes thinly and place in a shallow dish with the garlic and onion. Whisk the red wine vinegar and

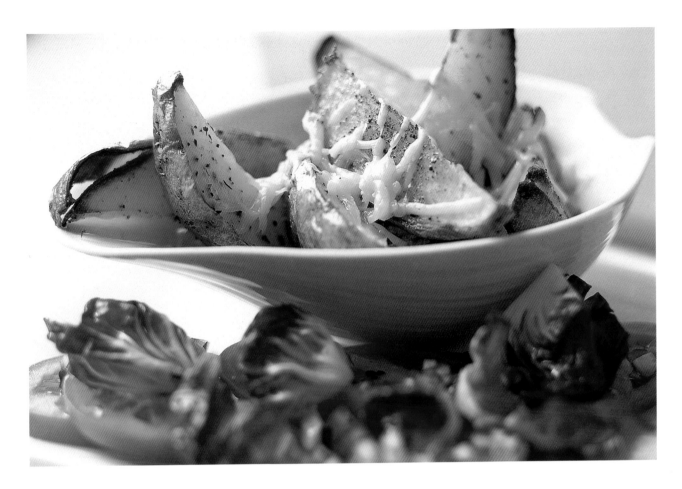

olive oil together, season to taste, then drizzle over the tomato salad. Set aside. Break the radicchio into small pieces, cover, and set aside.

5 Remove the potato wedges from the oven and turn the oven off. Arrange the slices of cheese over the wedges and return to the warm oven for 3–4 minutes, or until the cheese has melted.

6 Divide the potato wedges onto 4 serving plates with a large spoonful of the tomato and red onion salad and a large handful of the radicchio. Season with a grinding of pepper before serving.

HOMEMADE CAJUN SEASONING
If preferred, you can make your own Cajun seasoning. With a pestle and mortar, pound together 2 tablespoons (30 ml) ground paprika, 2 tablespoons (30 ml) cayenne pepper, 1 tablespoon (15 ml) black pepper, 2 tablespoons (30 ml) garlic granules, 2 tablespoons (30 ml) onion flakes, 1 tablespoon (15 ml) dried oregano, 1 tablespoon (15 ml) dried thyme, and 1 tablespoon (15 ml) salt, until you have a powdery consistency. This seasoning can be stored in an airtight jar for up to 3 months.

FOR THE SALAD

4 plum tomatoes

2 cloves garlic, peeled and finely chopped

I red onion, finely chopped

I tablespoon (15 ml) red wine vinegar

4 tablespoons (60 ml) extra virgin olive oil

Salt and pepper, to taste

I head radicchio

Serves 4

BACON & RICOTTA TART

1¼ cups (300 ml) sifted all-purpose flour, plus extra for dusting

1 level teaspoon (5 ml) instant yeast

1 level teaspoon (5 ml) salt

½ teaspoon (2 ml) sugar

1 tablespoon (15 ml) olive oil

2 cups (500 ml) ricotta cheese

⅔ cup (150 ml) sour cream

1 medium vidalia onion, thinly sliced

Salt and pepper, to taste

8 strips lean smoked bacon, roughly chopped

Olive oil, for drizzling

Serves 2–4

This makes a tasty meal when served with an arugula or spring mix salad. It is also perfect for a light lunch or picnic. If time is short, you could use a ready-made pizza base.

1   To make the dough, place the flour, yeast, salt and sugar in a warm bowl. Mix in the olive oil with ½ cup (125 ml) tepid water to make a soft dough. Knead the dough on a floured work surface for 3–4 minutes. Return the dough to the bowl, cover bowl with plastic wrap and leave in a warm place to rise for about 1 hour.

2   Meanwhile, to make the topping, mix the ricotta cheese, sour cream and onion together. Add a little salt and plenty of pepper. Preheat the oven to 450°F (230°C) and preheat a baking pan.

3   Once the dough has doubled in size, turn out onto a floured surface. Knead the dough for a couple of minutes to "knock out" the air. Shape the dough into a circle about 10 in (25 cm) in diameter.

4   Place the dough on the baking pan, spoon the ricotta mixture onto it, sprinkle with the bacon, and drizzle with olive oil. Cook for 20 minutes or until the bacon is crisp.

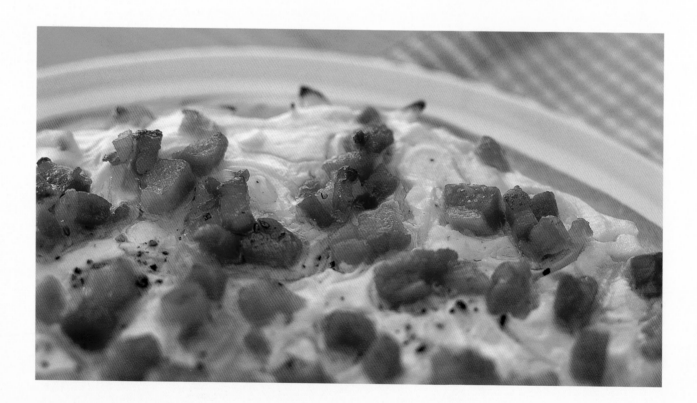

SWEET POTATO WITH COTTAGE CHEESE & CRISPY BACON

Cottage cheese is low in fat and still provides useful amounts of calcium. Adding a little crispy bacon helps to perk up its flavor.

1 Preheat the oven to 400°F (200°C). Pierce the potato in several places and wrap in foil. Bake in the oven for 45–60 minutes, or until soft.

2 Cook the bacon under a hot broiler until crispy. Chop into small pieces and mix into the cottage cheese.

3 Remove the potato from the foil and slice in half. Spoon the cottage cheese and bacon mixture onto it and serve.

1 medium sweet potato, about 9 oz (250 g)

2 strips lean smoked bacon

⅔ cup (175 ml) cottage cheese

Serves 1

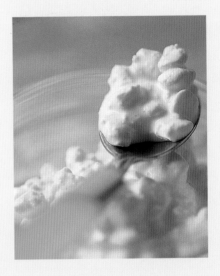

SPINACH & POTATO CAKE

Served with a simple tomato salad, this dish makes a healthy and satisfying lunch on a cold day.

1 Preheat the oven to 350°F (180°C). Melt the butter in a large saucepan, add the garlic and spinach, and cook until the spinach is just wilted. Drain well and chop roughly.

2 Mix together the spinach, eggs, crème fraîche or ricotta, milk, ½ cup (125 ml) of Gruyère cheese and the herbs. Season with salt, pepper, and nutmeg.

3 Lightly grease a 9-in (23-cm) springform cake pan. Cover the base with a layer of sliced potatoes, then a layer of the spinach mixture. Continue layering, finishing with layer of potatoes. Sprinkle with the remaining Gruyère cheese and cover the pan with lightly greased foil. Place in a roasting pan and pour in enough boiling water to reach halfway up the sides of the cake pan.

4 Bake for 1½ hours until the potatoes are tender—remove the foil for the last 15 minutes to allow the top to brown. Allow to cool in the pan for 5–10 minutes before serving.

1 tablespoon (15 ml) butter, plus extra for greasing

1 clove garlic, peeled and finely chopped

1 lb (500 g) fresh spinach, washed

3 eggs, beaten

1⅔ cups (400 ml) low-fat crème fraîche or ricotta cheese

2 tablespoons (30 ml) 2% milk

1¼ cups (300 ml) Gruyère or Swiss cheese, grated

3 tablespoons (45 ml) fresh mixed herbs, chopped

Salt and pepper, to taste

Pinch ground nutmeg

4 large potatoes, peeled and thinly sliced

Serves 6

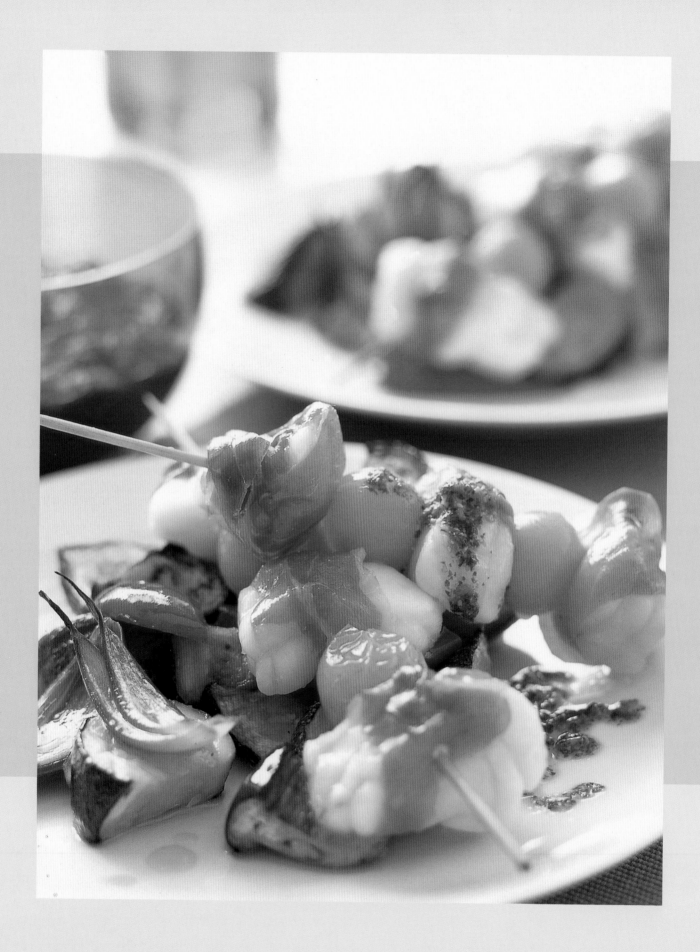

4

Main Courses

This chapter features meat, fish, and vegetarian main courses, ranging from those suitable for a quick family meal to ideas for a more elaborate dinner party. Most importantly, all the dishes provide essential vitamins and minerals for strong, healthy bones.

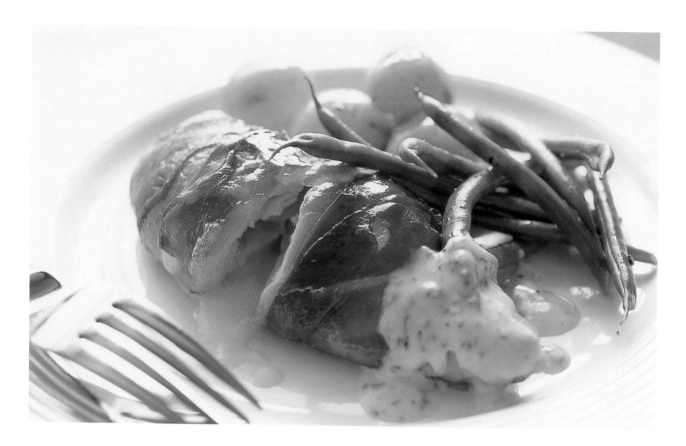

BRIE-STUFFED CHICKEN WITH CREAMY PESTO

4 boneless, skinless chicken breasts

7 oz (200 g) Brie

8 slices prosciutto

Vegetable oil, for frying

2 tablespoons (30 ml) green pesto

2 tablespoons (30 ml) Balkan-style yogurt

Serves 4

Mixing Balkan-style yogurt into the pesto gives it a wonderfully creamy flavor and helps to boost the calcium content of this dish. Serve with lightly steamed vegetables and new potatoes.

1 Cut sideways into each chicken breast to create a pocket. Cut the Brie into 4 slices and stuff one into each piece of chicken. Wrap 2 slices of prosciutto around each piece and secure with cocktail sticks.

2 Place the chicken on a lightly oiled baking tray and cook in the oven at 375°F (190°C) for 35 minutes, or until the chicken is cooked through.

3 Remove the cocktail sticks and transfer the chicken to a warm plate. Mix the pesto and yogurt together in a small bowl and drizzle the mixture over the cooked chicken.

FRESH PESTO

Place ½ cup (125 ml) fresh basil, 2 crushed cloves garlic, 2 tablespoons (30 ml) pine nuts, ½ cup (125 ml) olive oil and ½ cup (125 ml) freshly grated Parmesan cheese in a blender or food processor and purée until smooth. The fresh pesto will keep for up to 2 weeks in the fridge.

CHICKEN & WILD MUSHROOM STROGANOFF

Portobello and wild mushrooms can be found in supermarkets, but, if not, you can simply double the amount of button mushrooms. Serve with plain boiled rice or boiled new potatoes.

1 Cut the chicken into thin strips. Heat the butter and oil in a large deep nonstick frying pan or casserole dish until it foams. Add half the chicken and stir-fry over a high heat for 4–5 minutes until tender and lightly browned. Remove with a slotted spoon and drain on paper towel. Set aside. Repeat with the remaining chicken and set aside.

2 Add the onion, mushrooms, and red pepper to the frying pan or casserole dish and season well. Sauté over a medium heat for 5 minutes until the onion is soft. Add the tomato paste and cook for 1 minute. Add the stock and sour cream and stir well. Simmer for about 5 minutes until the mixture thickens slightly.

3 Return the chicken to the dish and simmer for 2–3 minutes to heat through. To serve, divide onto 4 warmed plates and sprinkle with snipped chives.

4 boneless, skinless chicken breasts

2 tablespoons (30 ml) butter

1 tablespoon (15 ml) olive oil

2 medium red onions, cut into wedges

¼ lb (125 g) button mushrooms, sliced

¼ lb (125 g) Portobello or wild mushrooms, sliced

1 red pepper, deseeded and sliced

Salt and pepper, to taste

2 tablespoons (30 ml) sun-dried tomato paste

1 cup (250 ml) chicken stock

⅔ cup (150 ml) sour cream

2 tablespoons (30 ml) fresh chives, snipped

Serves 4

GARLIC CHICKEN IN YOGURT

The yogurt and almonds boost the calcium content of this spiced chicken dish. Serve with plain boiled basmati rice.

1 Mix the chili flakes, cinnamon, 2 tablespoons (30 ml) olive oil, garlic, and curry paste together and season well. In a shallow dish, toss the chicken pieces with the curry paste mixture. Cover and leave for 20 minutes.

2 Heat the remaining oil in a large nonstick frying pan. Stir-fry the chicken for 4–5 minutes until tender and lightly browned.

3 Stir in the ground almonds and yogurt and heat through for 2–3 minutes. Sprinkle with the garam masala and cilantro and serve immediately.

1 teaspoon (5 ml) crushed chili flakes

1 teaspoon (5 ml) ground cinnamon

3 tablespoons (45 ml) olive oil

4 cloves garlic, peeled and finely crushed

2 teaspoons (10 ml) hot curry paste

Salt and pepper, to taste

¾ lb (350 g) boneless skinless chicken breast, cut into bite-sized pieces

1 cup (250 ml) ground almonds, toasted

1½ cups (325 ml) Balkan-style yogurt

1 teaspoon (5 ml) garam masala

2 tablespoons (30 ml) cilantro, chopped

Serves 4

CORONATION CHICKEN SALAD

Originally created for Queen Elizabeth II's coronation by the Cordon Bleu Cooking School, this is a more contemporary version. It is ideal for using up leftover cooked chicken, and makes a great sandwich filling.

FOR THE CHICKEN

¼ cup (50 ml) butter

1 medium onion, finely chopped

8 dried apricots, finely chopped

Small pinch saffron strands

Zest of 1 lemon

2 tablespoons (30 ml) liquid honey

2 tablespoons (30 ml) hot curry paste

⅞ cup (200 ml) dry white wine

8 tablespoons (120 ml) mayonnaise

8 tablespoons (120 ml) Balkan-style yogurt

1 lb (450 g) skinless, boneless cooked chicken, cut into bite-sized pieces

2 tablespoons (30 ml) chopped cilantro

Salt and pepper, to taste

FOR THE SALAD

1 sweet red pepper, thinly sliced

1 red chili, seeded and thinly sliced

4 green onions, cut into thin strips

½ cup (125 ml) unsalted peanuts, chopped

Arugula, to garnish

Cilantro sprigs, to garnish

Serves 4–6

1 Melt the butter in a saucepan and cook the onion for 5 minutes until soft. Add the apricots, saffron, lemon zest, honey, curry paste, and wine. Simmer uncovered for 25 minutes or until the mixture is the consistency of chutney or jam. Leave to cool.

2 Mix the mayonnaise with the yogurt, add the chicken and the cooled curry mixture and mix well. Add the cilantro and season to taste.

3 To make the salad, mix together the pepper, chili, green onions and peanuts. Divide the chicken onto 4–6 plates and top with the salad mixture. Serve with arugula leaves and more cilantro.

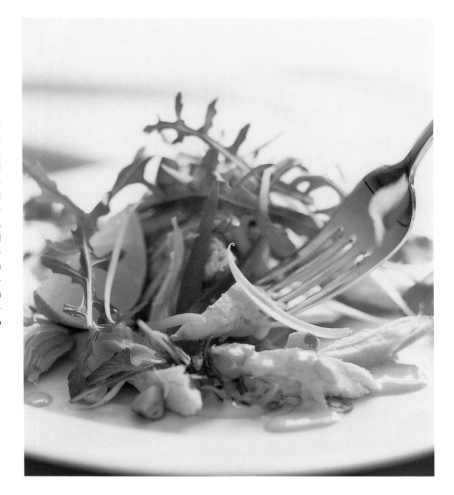

CHICKEN & SESAME BITES

Everyone will love these tasty little chicken bites. Sesame seeds have a deliciously nutty flavor and are a useful source of calcium, particularly for people who don't eat dairy products. Serve with a spicy tomato salsa.

1 Mix together the bread crumbs, sesame seeds, and seasoning, then spread over a large plate or baking tray.

2 Dip the chicken pieces into the beaten egg then roll in the bread crumb and sesame seed mixture until thoroughly coated. Carefully lay the chicken on a lightly greased baking sheet and place in the fridge for 30 minutes.

3 Meanwhile, preheat the oven to 400°F (200°C). Spray the chicken with olive oil and bake for 10–15 minutes, until the bread crumbs are golden brown and the chicken cooked through.

1½ cups (375 ml) fine white bread crumbs

⅓ cup (75 ml) sesame seeds

Salt and pepper, to taste

2 large skinless chicken breasts, cut into bite-sized pieces

1 egg, beaten

Extra virgin olive oil spray

Serves 4

QUICK TURKEY CASSOULET

This is a hearty and wholesome supper dish guaranteed to warm you up on a cold day. Turkey is a useful source of zinc, which is helpful in building strong bones. Serve with a crisp green salad.

1 Heat 2 tablespoons (30 ml) of the oil in a large nonstick saucepan. Add the onion, garlic, bacon and celery and cook over a low heat for 10 minutes, stirring occasionally.

2 Add the tomatoes, chicken stock, and soy sauce. Bring to a boil, then reduce to a fast simmer and cook for about 15 minutes, or until the sauce begins to thicken.

3 Add the mustard, beans, and turkey and continue to cook for a further 5 minutes. Transfer the mixture into a shallow ovenproof dish.

4 Mix the bread crumbs, Parmesan cheese, and parsley together and sprinkle over the turkey mixture. Drizzle with the remaining tablespoon of olive oil and place under a medium-hot broiler for 5 minutes, or until the bread crumbs are golden brown.

3 tablespoons (45 ml) olive oil

1 medium red onion, finely chopped

2 cloves garlic, crushed or finely chopped

¼ lb (125 g) smoked back bacon, roughly chopped

2 stalks celery, finely chopped

14 oz (400 g) can chopped tomatoes

1 cup (250 ml) chicken stock

2 tablespoons (30 ml) dark soy sauce

2 teaspoons (10 ml) Dijon mustard

2 14 oz (400 g) cans mixed beans, rinsed and drained

¾ lb (400 g) cooked turkey, roughly chopped

1½ cups (375 ml) fresh white bread crumbs

½ cup (125 ml) Parmesan cheese, freshly grated

3 tablespoons (45 ml) parsley, chopped

Serves 4

PORK STUFFED WITH APRICOTS & PINE NUTS

FOR THE STUFFING

1 tablespoon (15 ml) olive oil

1 medium onion, peeled and finely chopped

¾ cup (175 ml) fresh white bread crumbs

⅓ cup (75 ml) dried apricots, roughly chopped

¼ cup (50 ml) pine nuts, lightly toasted

2 tablespoons (30 ml) fresh parsley, chopped

Salt and pepper, to taste

1 small egg, beaten

FOR THE PORK

1 pork loin, about 2 lbs (900 g), trimmed

1 tablespoon (15 ml) olive oil

½ cup (125 ml) white wine

FOR THE GRAVY

2 teaspoons (10 ml) all-purpose flour

1⅔ cups (400 ml) chicken stock

3 tablespoons (45 ml) Balkan-style yogurt

1 tablespoon (15 ml) prepared mustard

Salt and pepper, to taste

Serves 4–6

Apricots are rich in potassium, which is beneficial for strong bones. They also provide useful amounts of calcium. Serve this for Sunday lunch with potatoes and green vegetables.

1 Preheat the oven to 350°F (180°C). To make the stuffing, heat the olive oil in a nonstick pan and fry the onion for 4–5 minutes until soft. In a large bowl, mix together the bread crumbs, apricots, pine nuts, parsley and seasoning. Add the cooked onion and the egg and mix well.

2 Split the pork almost in half, down the length of the loin, and spread the stuffing in the middle. Bring the two cut edges of pork together to enclose the stuffing and tie at intervals with string. Heat the oil in a pan, wait until it is hot, then add the pork and brown on all sides. Transfer the pork to a roasting pan, cut side down. Pour the wine over it and cook in the oven for 1 hour. Test that the pork is cooked by piercing the thickest part with a fine skewer—the juices should run clear. Transfer to a warm plate, cover with foil and keep warm while you make the gravy.

3 Put the roasting pan on the range and stir the flour into the juices from the meat. Gradually stir in the stock and simmer for 5 minutes, until the gravy begins to thicken. Stir in the yogurt and mustard and season to taste. Slice the pork and serve with the gravy.

PORK STUFFED WITH APPLE & WALNUTS

For an alternative stuffing, you can replace the apricots with ⅓ cup (75 ml) dried apple and the pine nuts with ¼ cup (50 ml) roughly chopped walnuts. To make the gravy, use 1 cup (250 ml) chicken stock and 1 cup (250 ml) dry cider.

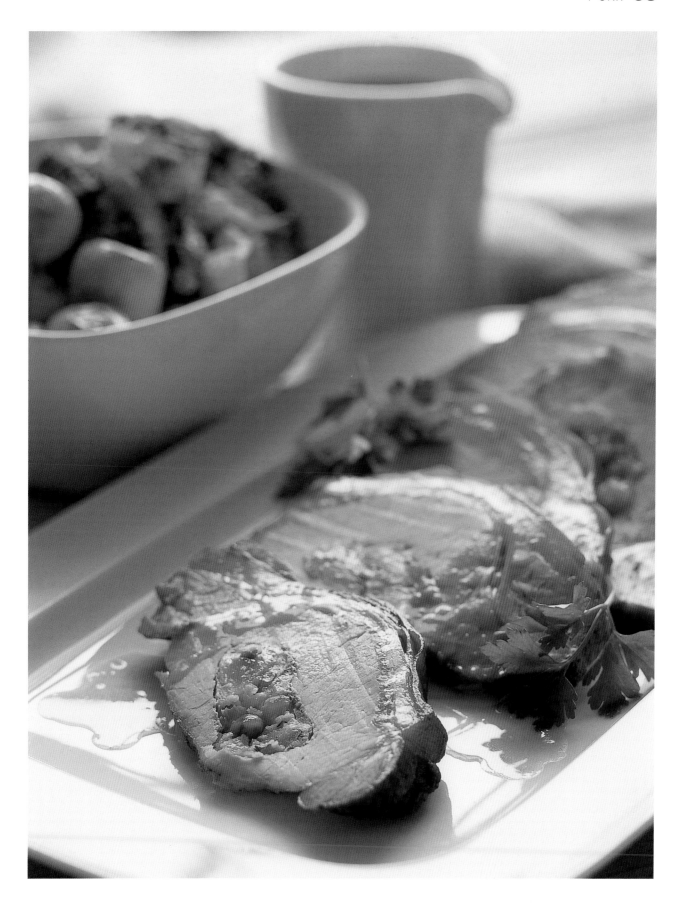

Pork with Bok Choy & Black Bean Sauce

Bok choy has a mild and pleasant flavor and a crisp texture. If you can't find bok choy, you can use Chinese cabbage instead.

2 tablespoons (30 ml) vegetable oil

1 lb (450 g) pork tenderloin, thinly sliced

2 cloves garlic, crushed or finely chopped

1 tablespoon (15 ml) fresh ginger, finely chopped

8 green onions, cut into ¼ in (0.5 cm) slices

¼ lb (125 g) shiitake mushrooms

½ lb (225 g) broccoli florets

4½ oz (125 g) baby corn, sliced lengthwise

¾ cup (175 ml) black bean sauce

1 tablespoon (15 ml) liquid honey

⅓ lb (150 g) bok choy, trimmed and sliced

2 cups (500 ml) egg noodles

1 tablespoon (15 ml) sesame oil

Green onions, thinly sliced, to garnish

Serves 4

1   Heat 1 tablespoon (15 ml) of the vegetable oil in a wok or large frying pan. Add the pork and stir-fry over a high heat for 5 minutes, or until browned. Remove from the pan and set aside.

2   Wipe the wok clean with paper towel and heat the remaining vegetable oil. Once the oil is hot, add the garlic, ginger, and green onions and stir-fry for 1 minute. Add the mushrooms, broccoli, and corn and continue cooking for 2–3 minutes.

3   Return the pork to the wok, stir in the black bean sauce, honey, bok choy, and ⅔ cup (150 ml) water. Cook for a further 5 minutes or until the sauce is hot.

4   Meanwhile, cook the noodles according to the package instructions. Drain well, then season with the sesame oil. To serve, place the noodles and pork stir-fry in a bowl and garnish with green onions.

Pork Escalopes with Celeriac Cream Mash

The dense texture of celeriac makes a delicious creamy mash, which provides an excellent accompaniment to plain meats, such as pork.

FOR THE MASH

1 lb (450 g) celeriac, peeled and cut into even-sized pieces

1 lb (450 g) potatoes, peeled and cut into even-sized pieces

1 tablespoon (15 ml) butter

3 green onions, finely chopped

⅔ cup (150 ml) crème fraîche or ricotta cheese

Salt and pepper, to taste

1   Bring a large pan of salted water to a boil. Add the celeriac and potato, bring back to a boil, and cook for 20–30 minutes, or until both are tender. Drain well, return to the pan, and mash.

2   In a small pan, heat the butter and cook the green onions for 2–3 minutes, until soft. Add the crème fraîche and warm through for 1 minute. Add the mixture to the mash, beat well, and season. Cover and keep warm until ready to serve.

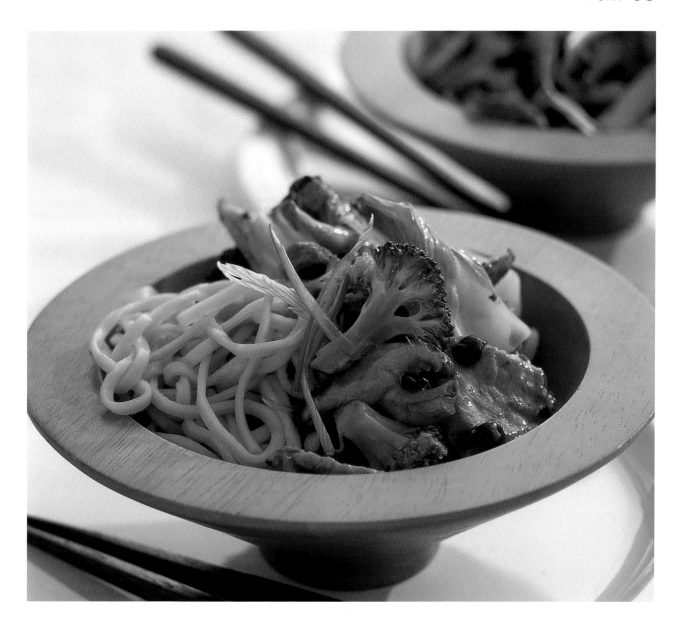

3 Meanwhile, put the escalopes between two sheets of waxed paper and thin by beating with a rolling pin. Brush each escalope with the melted butter and coat both sides with the bread crumbs.

4 Heat the broiler to medium. Arrange the breaded escalopes on a foil-lined broiler rack and broil for 3–4 minutes on each side.

5 Serve the escalopes on warm serving plates with a large spoonful of the celeriac mash. Garnish with sage leaves and freshly ground black pepper.

FOR THE ESCALOPES

4 pork escalopes, each
about ¼ lb (125 g)

2 tablespoons (30 ml) butter, melted

1 cup (250 ml) fine white bread crumbs

Fresh sage leaves, to garnish

Freshly ground black pepper

Serves 4

POLENTA WITH BACON & MUSHROOMS

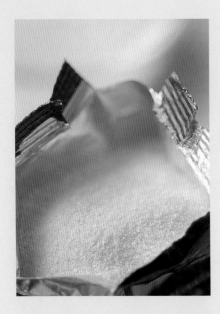

Polenta, which is made from cornmeal, is a speciality of northern Italy. For a change, you could replace the Parmesan with a blue cheese, such as Stilton, or goat cheese.

1 Place 3 cups (700 ml) of salted water in a large nonstick saucepan and bring to a boil. Pour in the cornmeal in a slow steady stream, stirring continuously. Reduce the heat and cook for 1 minute, or until the cornmeal is thick. Remove from the heat, stir in the Parmesan cheese, herbs, and butter and more salt, if required.

2 Spread the polenta into a shallow lightly oiled pan, to a thickness of about ½ in (1 cm). Allow to cool, then cut into triangles.

3 Heat the oil in a large nonstick frying pan. Add the bacon and cook over a high heat for 5 minutes, until it begins to brown. Add the green onions and mushrooms and continue to cook for a further 5 minutes. Add the stock, season to taste, and reduce the heat slightly. Cook for 20–30 minutes or until the liquid has reduced. Stir in the yogurt.

4 Place the polenta triangles under a preheated broiler for 3–4 minutes, turn, and continue to cook for a further 3 minutes. Transfer to warm plates, top with the bacon and mushroom mixture, and serve.

VEGETARIAN MUSHROOM POLENTA

This recipe can be adapted for vegetarians by simply omitting the bacon and using vegetable stock instead of chicken stock.

1¼ cups (300 ml) quick-cook cornmeal

1¼ cups (300 ml) Parmesan cheese, freshly grated

3 tablespoons (45 ml) fresh mixed herbs, roughly chopped

1 tablespoon (15 ml) butter

Salt, to taste

1 tablespoon (15 ml) olive oil

½ lb (225 g) rindless smoked back bacon, roughly chopped

8 green onions, chopped

⅔ lb (300 g) mixed mushrooms, roughly chopped

1¼ cups (300 ml) chicken stock

Salt and pepper, to taste

6 tablespoons (90 ml) Balkan-style yogurt

Serves 4

BROCCOLI & SMOKED HAM TAGLIATELLE

If you do not have fresh pasta, dried pasta can also be used in this dish —pasta shells work particularly well. Serve with a crisp green salad.

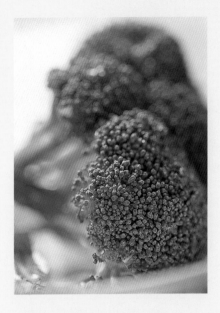

1 Cook the pasta in boiling salted water for 3–4 minutes, according to the package instructions, until *al dente*.

2 Meanwhile, melt the butter in a large saucepan, add the onion, broccoli and yellow pepper and fry for 5–7 minutes until just softened. Stir in the mascarpone cheese and heat through for 1–2 minutes until soft. Add the smoked ham, grated nutmeg, and flat-leaf parsley.

3 Fold the pasta into the sauce, season to taste, and heat through for 1–2 minutes. Heat the broiler to high. Turn the pasta into a shallow heatproof dish, sprinkle with Cheddar cheese, and broil until golden and bubbling.

VEGETABLE TAGLIATELLE
For a delicious vegetarian alternative, omit the ham and replace with ½ lb (225 g) mixture of any vegetables that can be cooked quickly, such as snow peas, mushrooms, or leeks.

8 oz (225 g) fresh green or white tagliatelle

2 tablespoons (30 ml) butter

1 large onion, halved and sliced

½ lb (225 g) small broccoli florets

1 yellow pepper, seeded and chopped

9 oz (250 g) mascarpone cheese

½ lb (225 g) smoked ham, shredded

½ teaspoon (2 ml) grated nutmeg

2 tablespoons (30 ml) flat-leaf parsley, chopped

Salt and pepper, to taste

1¼ cups (300 ml) Cheddar cheese, grated

Serves 4

Skewered Lamb with Tomato, Chili & Yogurt Marinade

FOR THE LAMB

1½ lbs (700 g) lamb neck fillet, trimmed and cut into chunks

1 tablespoon (15 ml) olive oil

2 cloves garlic, crushed

3 small red chilis, seeded and finely chopped

¼ cup (50 ml) sun-dried tomatoes in oil, drained and finely chopped

2 teaspoons (10 ml) balsamic vinegar

Pinch soft brown sugar

½ cup (125 ml) plain yogurt

Freshly ground black pepper, to taste

These tender marinated chunks of lamb are delicious served with basmati rice. Look out for small jars of chopped chilis in sunflower oil, as this speeds up the preparation and avoids the need to handle fresh chilis, which can be off-putting for some people.

1   Place the lamb, oil, garlic, chilis, sun-dried tomatoes, balsamic vinegar, brown sugar and yogurt together in a shallow bowl and stir well. Season with freshly ground black pepper. Cover, place in the fridge, and leave to marinate for at least 3 hours, or preferably overnight. Soak 4 wooden skewers in cold water for 30 minutes before using.

2   To make the rice, bring a large pan of water to a boil, stir in the rice, and add a pinch of salt. Return to a boil, cover and simmer for 12–14 minutes, or cook according to the package instructions. Drain well. Stir in the chopped cilantro and sun-dried tomatoes.

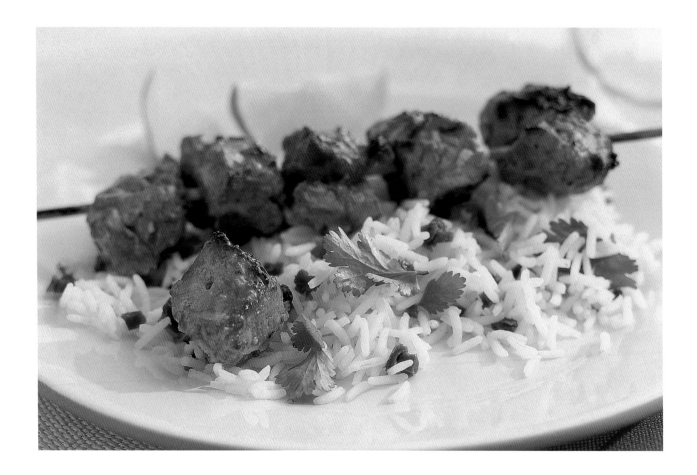

3 Heat the broiler to high. Thread the lamb onto the skewers, reserving the marinade. Put the skewered lamb on a broiler rack and broil for 3–4 minutes on each side for rare, or 5–6 minutes on each side for well done. Brush with the reserved marinade during broiling.

4 Serve the lamb on the skewers with the rice. Garnish with lime wedges and cilantro sprigs.

FOR THE RICE

1½ cups (375 ml) quick-cooking basmati rice

Pinch of salt

2 tablespoons (30 ml) cilantro, chopped

1 tablespoon (15 ml) sun-dried tomatoes in oil, drained and finely chopped

Lime wedges, to garnish

Cilantro sprigs, to garnish

Serves 4

GARLIC & CUMIN ROASTED LAMB WITH APRICOT & CHICKPEA SALSA

Here, roast lamb is given an unusual twist when served with a tangy salsa. The salsa can be made in advance and stored, covered, in the fridge until ready to serve—remove from the fridge while cooking the lamb to allow the flavors to develop.

1 Preheat the oven to 400°F (200°C). Rub the cumin seeds over the lamb fillets. Using a small sharp knife, make small cuts all over the fillets and insert the garlic slivers.

2 Put the lamb fillets into a roasting pan and roast in the oven for 30 minutes, until tender.

3 Meanwhile, make the salsa. Combine the red onion, chili, sun-dried tomatoes, apricots, chickpeas, oil, lime zest and juice, and cilantro together in a bowl. Cover and set aside.

4 When the lamb is cooked, remove from the oven and leave to stand for 5 minutes. To serve, slice the lamb and top with the salsa. Garnish with mint leaves.

1 teaspoon (5 ml) cumin seeds

6 lamb neck fillets

2 garlic cloves, cut into slivers

FOR THE SALSA

1 small red onion, finely chopped

1 red chili, seeded and finely chopped

2 sun-dried tomatoes, finely chopped

1 cup (250 ml) dried apricots, finely chopped

14 oz (400 g) can chickpeas, drained and rinsed

1 tablespoon (15 ml) olive oil

Zest and juice of 1 lime

1 tablespoon (15 ml) cilantro, chopped

Fresh mint leaves, to garnish

Serves 4

MOROCCAN LAMB WITH CHICKPEAS & APRICOTS

2 teaspoons (10 ml) ground ginger

2 teaspoons (10 ml) ground cumin

2 teaspoons (10 ml) paprika

1 cinnamon stick

Scant ½ cup (125 ml) orange juice

1 lb (450 g) lamb stew, cut into
bite-sized pieces

1 tablespoon (15 ml) vegetable oil

8 shallots or pearl onions, peeled

2 cloves garlic, peeled and crushed

1 tablespoon (15 ml) all-purpose flour

1 tablespoon (15 ml) tomato paste

1 cup (250 ml) chicken stock

⅔ cup (150 ml) sherry

Salt and pepper, to taste

1 cup (250 ml) dried apricots

14 oz (400 g) can chickpeas,
drained and rinsed

Cilantro, chopped, to garnish

Serves 4

*Here, the lamb is marinated in a tangy, spicy marinade, which gives
it a delicious flavor. Both chickpeas and apricots are good sources
of calcium, so this dish is great for people on dairy-free diets.
Serve with couscous or plain rice.*

1 Put the ginger, cumin, paprika, and the cinnamon stick in a large bowl and pour on the orange juice. Add the lamb and mix well. Cover and leave in a cool place for at least 1 hour, or preferably overnight.

2 Preheat the oven to 350°F (180°C). Heat the oil in a large flameproof casserole dish. Remove the lamb from the marinade and cook it in the dish over a high heat for 5 minutes until lightly browned. Remove with a slotted spoon and set aside.

3 Lower the heat and add a little more oil if necessary. Cook the onions and garlic for 3 minutes, or until they are just beginning to brown. Return the lamb to the dish, stir in the flour and tomato paste and continue cooking for 1 minute, stirring frequently.

4 Add the remaining marinade, stock, and sherry and season to taste. Bring to a boil then reduce the heat, cover, and bake in the oven for 1 hour.

5 Add the apricots and chickpeas and return to the oven for a further 15 minutes. Garnish with chopped cilantro and serve.

MOROCCAN LAMB WITH FAVA BEANS & PRUNES
For a change, try replacing the chickpeas with canned fava beans and the apricots with prunes.

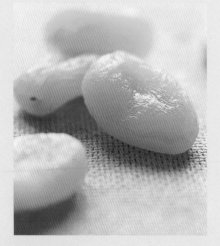

MOUSSAKA

The combination of ricotta, Parmesan and Cheddar cheeses makes this warm and comforting dish a real calcium booster. Choose lean ground lamb to help reduce the fat content. Serve with a mixed green salad.

1 Preheat the oven to 350°F (180°C). Heat 1 tablespoon (15 ml) of the oil in a nonstick saucepan, add the onion and garlic, and fry for 5 minutes, or until soft.

2 Add the lamb and cook until tender and browned. Add the tomatoes, tomato paste, cinnamon, oregano, and seasoning. Bring to a boil and cook over a low heat for about 20 minutes.

3 Place the potato in a large pan of boiling salted water and cook for 5 minutes. Drain well. Brush the eggplant with the remaining oil and place under a hot broiler for 4 minutes on each side, until nicely browned.

4 Mix together the ricotta and Parmesan cheeses. Stir in the beaten egg and milk and season to taste.

5 Arrange half of the broiled eggplant over the base of a shallow ovenproof dish. Add a layer of meat sauce, cover with the remaining eggplant and top with the sliced potatoes.

6 Pour the cheese sauce on the top, sprinkle with the Cheddar cheese, and bake in the oven for 30–40 minutes.

2 tablespoons (30 ml) olive oil

I large red onion, peeled and finely chopped

2 cloves garlic, crushed or finely chopped

I lb (450 g) lean ground lamb

28 oz (800 g) canned chopped tomatoes

I tablespoon (15 ml) sun-dried tomato paste

¼ teaspoon (I ml) ground cinnamon

I teaspoon (5 ml) dried oregano

Salt and pepper, to taste

I large potato, peeled and thinly sliced

I large eggplant, cut into slices ¼ in (0.5 cm) thick

9 oz (250 g) ricotta cheese

½ cup (125 ml) fresh Parmesan cheese, grated

I egg, beaten

4 tablespoons (60 ml) whole milk

¼ cup (50 ml) Cheddar cheese, grated

Serves 4

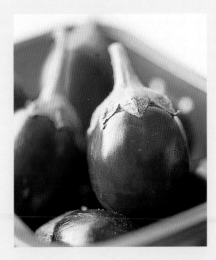

SHEPHERD'S PIE

1 lb (450 g) ground lamb

1 large onion, chopped

1 bay leaf

½ cup (125 ml) mushrooms, sliced

2 medium carrots, sliced

2 tablespoons (30 ml) all-purpose flour

1¼ cups (300 ml) stewed tomatoes, chopped

1 tablespoon (15 ml) sun-dried tomato paste

Salt and pepper, to taste

1½ lbs (700 g) potatoes, peeled and cut into even-sized pieces

2 tablespoons (30 ml) butter

4 tablespoons (60 ml) whole milk

¾ cup (175 ml) white crumbly cheese, such as goat milk cheese

Serves 4

This version has more flavorsome ingredients than many traditional shepherd's pie recipes and has a delicious cheese topping. Serve with a steamed green vegetable, such as broccoli.

1 Sauté the ground lamb with the onion, bay leaf, mushrooms and carrots for 8–10 minutes.

2 Add the flour and cook, stirring, for 1 minute. Gradually blend in the stewed tomatoes and tomato paste. Cook, stirring, until the mixture thickens and boils. Cover and simmer gently for 25 minutes.

3 Remove the bay leaf and season to taste. Spoon into an ovenproof dish.

4 Heat the oven to 400°F (200°C). Cook the potatoes in boiling salted water for 20 minutes, until tender. Drain well and mash with the butter and milk. Spread the mashed potato over the ground-meat mixture and sprinkle with the crumbled cheese. Bake for 15–20 minutes until golden brown.

BLUE CHEESE & WALNUT STEAKS

1¼ cups (300 ml) Stilton or other blue cheese, crumbled

2 tablespoons (30 ml) butter, softened

½–¾ cup (125–175 ml) walnut pieces, finely chopped

Freshly ground black pepper, to taste

4 sirloin steaks, each weighing about 4–6 oz (125–180 g), trimmed

Serves 4

These steaks have a tasty, and unexpectedly crunchy, topping. Simple accompaniments, such as boiled potatoes and a mixed salad, are all that are needed to complete this meal.

1 Put the cheese in a bowl and mash with a fork. Add butter and walnuts and mix thoroughly. Season to taste with pepper.

2 Preheat the broiler to high. Put the steaks on a broiler rack and season with plenty of pepper. Place under the broiler and cook for 1–2 minutes on each side for rare, 4 minutes on each side for medium, and 6–7 minutes on each side for well done.

3 Remove the steaks from under the broiler and sprinkle with the cheese and nut mixture. Press down the mixture with a palette knife. Broil for 1 minute, or until the topping is melted and bubbling. Serve hot.

MEATBALLS WITH MOZZARELLA & TOMATO SAUCE

The mozzarella cheese melts while the meatballs are cooking to give a deliciously creamy filling. Combined with a rich tomato sauce, this makes a comforting supper, when served with a large plate of spaghetti.

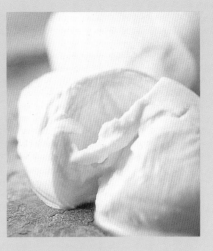

1   To make the meatballs, heat the olive oil in a large nonstick pan. Add the onion and the garlic and cook over a low heat for 5 minutes, until soft. Place the ground beef, bread crumbs, egg, and Parmesan cheese in a bowl. Add the cooked onions and garlic and mix well.

2   Cut or tear the mozzarella cheese into 20 small pieces. Take a heaping tablespoon of the ground-meat mixture and shape into a ball around a piece of mozzarella cheese. Repeat the process with the remaining meat, until you have 20 meatballs. Place the meatballs on a plate or tray and chill for 30 minutes.

3   To make the sauce, heat the oil in a saucepan, add the onion and cook for 4–5 minutes. Add the garlic, tomatoes, tomato paste, mixed herbs, red wine, and seasoning. Bring to a boil, reduce the heat, cover, and simmer over a low heat for 15 minutes, stirring occasionally. Remove the lid, add the meatballs, and continue to cook for a further 20 minutes. Serve the meatballs covered with the sauce.

FOR THE MEATBALLS

1 tablespoon (15 ml) olive oil

½ small onion, finely chopped

½ clove garlic, peeled and finely chopped

1 lb (450 g) lean ground beef

1 cup (250 ml) fine white bread crumbs

1 egg, beaten

2 tablespoons (30 ml) Parmesan cheese, freshly grated

¾ cup (175 ml) mozzarella cheese

FOR THE SAUCE

1 tablespoon (15 ml) olive oil

½ small onion, finely chopped

½ clove garlic, peeled and finely chopped

28 oz (800 g) canned chopped tomatoes

1 tablespoon (15 ml) tomato paste

1 teaspoon (5 ml) dried mixed herbs

⅔ cup (150 ml) red wine

Salt and pepper, to taste

Serves 4

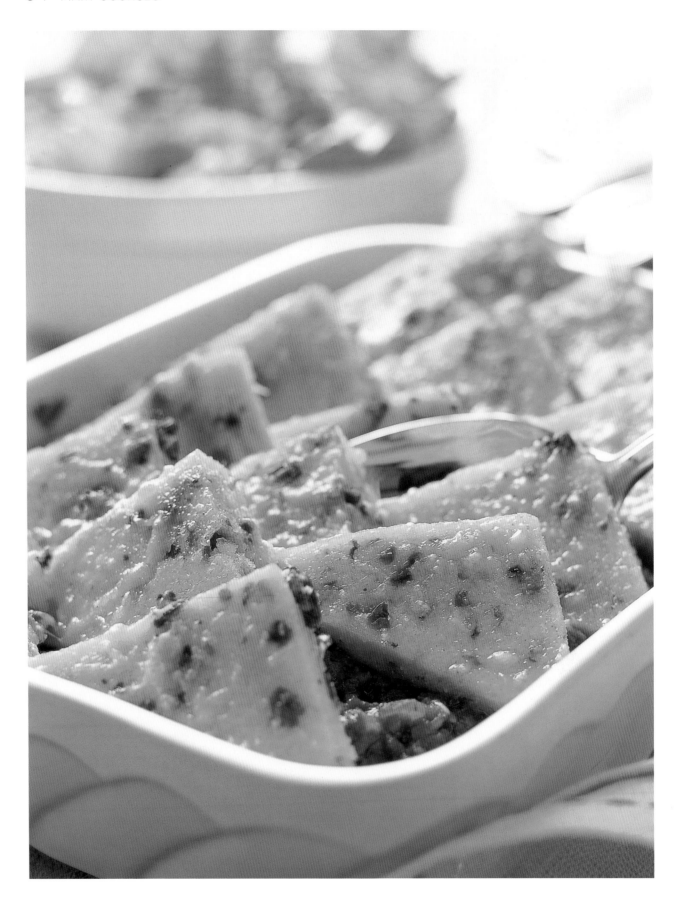

GROUND BEEF WITH POLENTA TOPPING

Polenta is gluten-free, so this is a good alternative to a pastry-topped pie for anyone who can't eat wheat or gluten. Mixing Parmesan cheese with the polenta helps boost both the flavor and the calcium content. Serve with a green salad.

1 Heat the oil in large nonstick saucepan. Add the onion and garlic and cook for 5 minutes until soft. Add the beef and cook until browned.

2 Stir in the tomatoes, tomato paste, wine and seasoning and bring to a boil. Reduce the heat and simmer gently for 30 minutes.

3 To make the polenta topping, place 3 cups (700 ml) of salted water in a large saucepan and bring to a boil. Pour in the cornmeal in a slow steady stream, stirring continuously. Reduce the heat to low and cook for 1 minute or until the polenta is thick. Stir in the Parmesan cheese, the sun-dried tomatoes, rosemary and butter and add more salt, if required. Spread the polenta into a shallow lightly oiled pan, to a thickness of about ½ in (1 cm). Allow to cool.

4 Once the polenta is cold, cut it into triangles. Heat the oven to 400°F (200°C). Place the beef mixture in a shallow ovenproof dish and arrange the polenta over the top so that the triangles overlap slightly.

5 Sprinkle with Parmesan cheese and bake at for 20–30 minutes, until the topping is golden brown.

OLIVE AND BLUE CHEESE POLENTA TOPPING
Adding different flavors to the polenta topping transforms this recipe. Add ¼ cup (50 ml) pitted, roughly chopped black olives to the polenta and use 1¼ cups (300 ml) crumbled blue cheese, such as Stilton, instead of the Parmesan.

1 tablespoon (15 ml) olive oil

1 medium red onion, peeled and finely chopped

1 large clove garlic, finely chopped

1 lb (450 g) lean ground beef

28 oz (800 g) canned chopped tomatoes

2 tablespoons (30 ml) sun-dried tomato paste

1 cup (250 ml) red wine

Salt and pepper, to taste

FOR THE POLENTA TOPPING

1 cup (250 ml) quick-cook cornmeal

¾ cup (175 ml) Parmesan cheese, freshly grated, plus extra for sprinkling

¾ cup (175 ml) sun-dried tomatoes, roughly chopped

½ teaspoon (2 ml) fresh rosemary, chopped

1 tablespoon (15 ml) butter

Salt, to taste

Vegetable oil, for greasing

Serves 4

SALMON FISH CAKES

1¼ lbs (550 g) potatoes, peeled and cut into large chunks

2 tablespoons (30 ml) mayonnaise

15 oz (418 g) can salmon, drained

Salt and pepper, to taste

All-purpose flour, for dusting

1 large egg, beaten

2 cups (500 ml) fine white bread crumbs

¼ cup (50 ml) sunflower oil

Lemon wedges, to garnish

Serves 4

Nutritionists recommend that we eat at least two servings of oil-rich fish, such as salmon, a week. As well as providing healthy omega-3 fatty acids, canned salmon, when eaten with the bones, is an excellent source of calcium. Serve the fish cakes with tzatziki and new potatoes.

1 Place the potatoes in a large pan of salted water, bring to a boil, and cook for about 20 minutes, until tender. Drain well and mash with the mayonnaise.

2 Place the salmon, including the bones, in a large bowl and mash with a fork. Add the mashed potato and season to taste. Mix well, then cover and place in the fridge for 1 hour.

3 Remove the mixture from the fridge. Shape into 8 fish cakes and dust with flour. Carefully dip each fish cake into the beaten egg, then into the bread crumbs, making sure it is evenly coated.

4 Heat half the oil in a large nonstick frying pan and cook half the fish cakes over a high heat for 4 minutes each side, until the bread crumbs are golden brown. Drain on absorbent paper towel, then transfer to a warm oven while you cook the remaining fish cakes. Garnish with lemon wedges.

SALMON & LEEK LASAGNA

2 tablespoons (30 ml) butter

2 large leeks, washed and thinly sliced

¼ cup (50 ml) all-purpose flour

2½ cups (600 ml) 2% milk

2¼ cups (550 ml) Cheddar cheese, grated

Salt and pepper, to taste

7.5-oz (225 g) can salmon, drained and flaked

8 lasagna noodles, cooked and drained

2 tablespoons (30 ml) sunflower seeds, toasted

Serves 4

Canned salmon provides a useful source of calcium, vitamin D, and phosphorus, all of which are essential for strong bones. Serve this lasagna with a large green salad and crusty bread.

1 Preheat the oven to 375˚F (190°C). Grease a shallow ovenproof dish.

2 Heat the butter in a large nonstick frying pan, add the leeks, and cook for 4–5 minutes until soft.

3 Place the flour and milk in a small saucepan, whisk together, then slowly bring to a boil, stirring continuously. Reduce the heat and simmer for 1 minute. Remove from the heat, stir in half of the cheese, and season to taste.

4 Mix the leeks, half of the cheese sauce, and the salmon together. Spoon half the salmon and leek mixture into the bottom of the prepared dish and top with a layer of lasagna. Make a layer with the remaining salmon mixture, top with a final layer of lasagna, and cover with the remaining cheese sauce. Sprinkle with the remaining cheese and the sunflower seeds. Bake in the oven for 20 minutes, until the top is bubbling.

SMOKED SALMON & DILL QUICHE

The sweet aniseed flavor of the dill complements the smoked salmon perfectly in this nourishing, creamy dish.

1   Roll out the pastry on a lightly floured surface and use to line a 9-in (23-cm) loose-bottomed, 1½-in (4-cm) deep, flan pan. Place on a baking sheet, cover and chill in the fridge for 30 minutes. Preheat the oven to 400°F (200°C).

2   Prick the base of the flan, line with a large sheet of baking parchment or foil paper and fill with dried beans. Bake for 10–15 minutes, then carefully remove the paper and the beans. Return to the oven for a further 5 minutes until the base is firm to the touch and lightly golden. Remove from the oven and set aside while making the filling.

3   Heat the oil and cook the onion for 5 minutes until soft. Turn down the oven to 325°F (170°C). Chop the fresh dill, reserving several sprigs to garnish. Whisk the eggs and cheeses together until smooth, then whisk in the cream, dill, and pepper. Scatter the onion and salmon over the base of the crust and pour in the egg mixture.

4   Bake the quiche for 45–55 minutes, until lightly set. Garnish with smoked salmon trimmings and dill sprigs.

½ lb (225 g) ready-made shortcrust pastry or pie shell

All-purpose flour, for dusting

1 tablespoon (15 ml) oil

1 large onion, finely chopped

2 eggs

7 oz (200 g) soft cream cheese

1 oz (25 g) rindless soft goat cheese

1¼ cups (300 ml) light cream

1 tablespoon (15 ml) fresh dill, plus extra to garnish

Pepper, to taste

¼ lb (125 g) smoked salmon, roughly chopped, plus extra to garnish

Serves 6

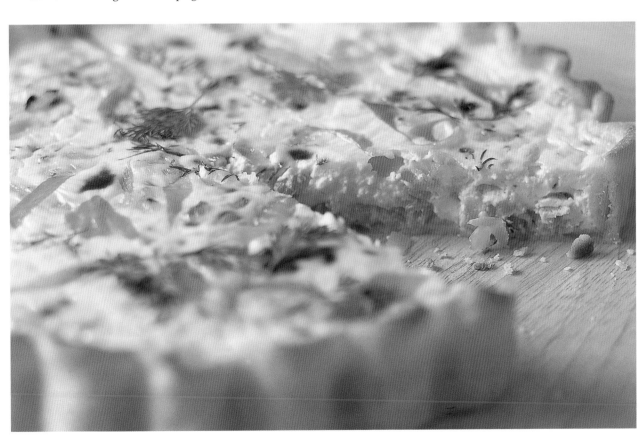

Quick Salmon Kedgeree

1½ cups (375 ml) basmati rice

2 teaspoons (30 ml) olive oil

4 green onions, roughly chopped

7.5 oz (225 g) can salmon, drained, bones and skin removed, then roughly flaked

½ teaspoon (2 ml) coriander seeds, finely crushed

3 tablespoons (45 ml) heavy cream

3 hard-boiled eggs, quartered

3 tablespoons (45 ml) fresh parsley, plus extra to garnish

Salt and pepper, to taste

2 lemons, cut into wedges, to garnish

Serves 4

Oil-rich fish, such as salmon, are one of the few dietary sources of vitamin D, which is essential for the absorption of calcium. This delicious rice dish is ideal for brunch.

1 Bring a large pan of boiling salted water to a boil. Stir in the rice and return to a boil, then cover and simmer for 12–14 minutes until just tender. Drain the rice well, rinse with boiling water, and drain again.

2 Meanwhile, heat the oil in a large nonstick frying pan and cook the green onions for 1–2 minutes until soft.

3 Chop the parsley, reserving several springs to garnish. Add the cooked rice, salmon, coriander seeds, cream, hard-boiled eggs, and chopped parsley. Season lightly and heat through gently for 2 minutes.

4 Spoon the kedgeree onto warmed serving plates and garnish with the lemon wedges, flat-leaf parsley sprigs, and a grinding of black pepper.

TUNA KEDGEREE
This kedgeree can also be made with tuna. Replace the salmon with 7½ oz (213 g) canned tuna in sunflower oil—drain and flake the tuna before using.

Salmon with a Crumb Crust

1 cup (250 ml) fine white bread crumbs

1 tablespoon (15 ml) pine nuts, lightly toasted

4 tablespoons (60 ml) fresh basil, chopped

1 tablespoon (15 ml) butter

½ cup (125 ml) Parmesan cheese, freshly grated

Salt and pepper, to taste

4 salmon steaks

Serves 4

This recipe is quick and easy and is an ideal dish for a quick midweek supper party—serve with new potatoes and green beans.

1 Heat the broiler. Place the bread crumbs, pine nuts, basil, butter, Parmesan cheese, and seasoning in a food processor and blend until combined.

2 Place the salmon under a moderately hot broiler for 5 minutes. Turn over, top with the bread crumb mixture, pressing it down gently with the palm of your hand. Broil for a further 5 minutes, or until the salmon is cooked through.

COD & BROCCOLI CHEESE PIE

Here, chunks of fish are cooked in a creamy cheese sauce, under a layer of golden cheese and mashed potato. Using mascarpone cheese is a quick way to make a cheese sauce and is a good source of calcium.

1 Preheat the oven to 350°F (180°C). Place the cod in an ovenproof dish and cover with 2 cups (450 ml) of the milk. Add the onion, carrot, and the bay leaf. Cover and cook in the oven for 20 minutes. Strain off, and discard, the milk.

2 Meanwhile, cook the potatoes in boiling water for 20 minutes. Drain and return to the saucepan. Add 2 tablespoons (30 ml) of the butter and mash smoothly. Add the cream and the remaining milk and beat until light and fluffy. Season well, then fold in half the Cheddar cheese.

3 In the meantime, blanch the broccoli in boiling salted water for 1 minute. Drain well and rinse under cold running water. Set aside on a plate lined with paper towel.

4 Melt 2 tablespoons (30 ml) of the butter in a saucepan and cook the leeks for 5–7 minutes, until softened. Add the mascarpone and stir well until smooth. Cook for 5–7 minutes until thickened. Chop the dill, reserving several springs to garnish. Stir the dill into the mascarpone and season well.

5 Turn the oven up to 450°F (230°C). Flake the cod in the ovenproof dish, place the broccoli evenly over the flaked fish, then pour on the sauce. Add the mashed potato, covering the filling completely, and sprinkle with the remaining Cheddar cheese. Dot with the remaining butter and bake in the oven for 10–15 minutes until brown on top. Serve garnished with sprigs of fresh dill.

1½ lbs (750 g) cod fillet

2½ cups (600 ml) whole milk

½ onion, sliced

1 carrot, thinly sliced

1 bay leaf

2 lbs (1 kg) potatoes, peeled and cut into even-sized pieces

6 tablespoons (90 ml) butter

⅔ cup (150 ml) light cream

Salt and pepper, to taste

1 cup (250 ml) old Cheddar cheese, grated

½ lb (225 g) small broccoli florets

1 large leek, thinly sliced

1¼ lbs (500 g) mascarpone cheese

1 tablespoon (15 ml) fresh dill, plus extra to garnish

Serves 6

SALMON AND BROCCOLI CHEESE PIE

Replace the fresh cod with 1½ lbs (750 g) fresh salmon. Flavor the mashed potato with some finely chopped green onions or chopped fresh herbs, such as dill, tarragon, or chervil.

PARSNIP TOPPING

Replace half of the potatoes with parsnips to make a parsnip mash topping, then follow the recipe as above.

CARROT TOPPING

For a potato and carrot topping, use 1½ lbs (750 g) potato and fold 1¼ cups (300 ml) grated carrot into the mash, then follow the recipe as above.

COD BAKED IN YOGURT

⅔ cup (150 ml) plain yogurt

1 clove garlic, peeled and finely chopped

1 tablespoon (15 ml) ginger root, finely chopped

½ teaspoon (2 ml) ground cumin

½ teaspoon (2 ml) ground coriander

¼ teaspoon (1 ml) chili powder

¼ teaspoon (1 ml) salt

4 skinless cod fillets

Serves 4

This dish is low in fat, making it a good choice for anyone on a weight-reducing or low-fat diet. If you haven't got the individual spices at hand, you could use 1 tablespoon (15 ml) of curry paste instead. Serve the fish with a tomato salad and naan bread.

1 Mix together the yogurt, garlic, ginger, cumin, coriander, chili and salt.

2 Place the fish in a shallow dish and pour the spiced yogurt mixture over it. Cover and refrigerate for 2–3 hours.

3 Heat the broiler. Transfer the fish onto a foil-lined broiler pan and cook under a hot broiler for 5–8 minutes, or until the fish is cooked through.

POACHED HADDOCK WITH SPINACH & POACHED EGG

2 smoked haddock steaks, about 6 oz (150 g) each

⅔ cup (150 ml) whole milk

2 large eggs

1¾ cups (425 ml) baby spinach leaves, washed and drained

Salt and pepper, to taste

Serves 2

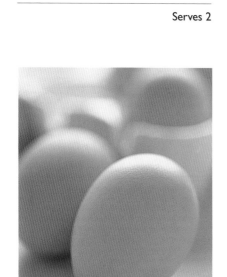

This dish makes a healthy and nutritious lunch or light supper. Spinach provides useful amounts of calcium, particularly for people who don't eat dairy products. Egg yolks are rich in vitamin K, which is essential for bone health.

1 Place the haddock in a large shallow pan and pour the milk over it. Cover and simmer gently for about 8 minutes, or until cooked through.

2 Meanwhile, bring a pan of water to a boil, then carefully crack the eggs into the water and poach for 2–3 minutes. Remove with a slotted spoon, allowing the water to drain thoroughly. Set aside on plate lined with paper towel.

3 Cook the spinach in a large saucepan for 2–3 minutes until just wilted— there is no need to add extra water as enough clings to the leaves after washing. Season well.

4 Divide the spinach onto two plates and place a haddock steak on top of the spinach. Top each with a poached egg.

FISH PIE WITH RÖSTI TOPPING

A crisp potato and red onion topping hides a rich creamy mixture of smoked haddock, small peas, and green beans.

1   Cook the potatoes, whole, in their skins, in plenty of boiling salted water for 15 minutes. Drain well and set aside to cool.

2   Meanwhile, heat the oil in a saucepan and cook the onion for 5–7 minutes, until soft and lightly golden. Peel and coarsely grate the potatoes into a sieve, squeezing out any excess moisture. Mix the potatoes, onion, and chopped herbs together and season well. Set aside.

3   Put the haddock, peppercorns and stock in a large pan. Bring to a boil, then cover and simmer gently for about 5–7 minutes, or until the fish is just tender. Remove the fish from the stock and flake the flesh, discarding the skin and any bones. Set aside.

4   Cook the peas and French beans in boiling salted water for 4–5 minutes, or until just tender. Drain well.

5   Heat the oven to 400°F (200°C). In a saucepan, gently heat the mascarpone and cook for 5–7 minutes until it has thickened. Put the fish, peas, and green beans in a shallow ovenproof dish and pour over the cheese sauce. Gently mix and season to taste.

6   Mix the potato and onion with the melted butter and spoon over the fish mixture, making sure it covers the filling. Cook in the oven for 20–25 minutes, until golden brown.

FOR THE TOPPING

1½ lbs (750 g) large waxy potatoes

2 tablespoons (30 ml) olive oil

1 large red onion, thinly sliced

1 tablespoon (15 ml) fresh mixed herbs, chopped

Salt and pepper, to taste

FOR THE FILLING

1 lb (450 g) smoked haddock

6 whole peppercorns

1 cup (250 ml) fish or vegetable stock

¼ lb (125 g) frozen small peas

¼ lb (125 g) green beans, halved

1¼ lbs (500 g) mascarpone cheese

Salt and pepper, to taste

2 tablespoons (30 ml) melted butter

Serves 6

DEEP-FRIED SMELT

Like all fish that are eaten with their bones, smelt are an excellent source of calcium. Mixing a little plain yogurt with the mayonnaise helps to reduce the fat content and boost the calcium content.

1   Mix the paprika with the flour and season to taste. Toss the smelt in the seasoned flour.

2   Heat the oil in a deep fat fryer to 375°F (190°C). Add the smelt to the hot oil in batches, cooking each batch for about 3 minutes, until the fish is golden brown. Drain on paper towel and keep warm while you cook the rest.

3   Mix the mayonnaise, yogurt, chives, and lemon zest together. Garnish the smelt with lemon wedges and serve with the yogurt dip.

1 tablespoon (15 ml) paprika

6 tablespoons (90 ml) all-purpose flour

Salt and pepper, to taste

1 lb (450 g) smelt

Oil, for deep-frying

5 tablespoons (75 ml) mayonnaise

3 tablespoons (45 ml) plain yogurt

2 tablespoons (30 ml) chopped chives

Zest of 1 lemon

Lemon wedges, to garnish

Serves 4

MONKFISH KABOBS WITH ROASTED VEGETABLES & PESTO

FOR THE ROASTED VEGETABLES

2 red peppers, seeded and cut into bite-sized pieces

1 large eggplant, cut into bite-sized pieces

2 small red onions, peeled and cut into quarters

2 large zucchini, sliced into bite-sized pieces

6 cloves garlic, peeled

4 tablespoons (60 ml) olive oil

Salt and pepper, to taste

FOR THE PESTO

1 cup (250 ml) fresh watercress, chopped

1 clove garlic, peeled

½ cup (125 ml) Parmesan cheese, freshly grated

6 tablespoons (90 ml) olive oil

FOR THE KABOBS

1 lb (450 g) monkfish, cut into 24 bite-sized pieces

6 slices prosciutto, cut into strips

16 cherry tomatoes

Serves 4

Using watercress instead of basil in the pesto helps to boost the calcium content. Watercress is also rich in vitamin C and beta carotene, and provides useful amounts of iron.

1 Preheat the oven to 425°F (220°C). Place the red peppers, eggplant, onions, zucchini and garlic in a large roasting pan, drizzle with the olive oil, and mix well. Season and place in the oven for 20–30 minutes, until the vegetables are tender.

2 To make the pesto, place the watercress, garlic, Parmesan cheese, and olive oil in a blender or food processor and blend until smooth.

3 Wrap each piece of monkfish in a strip of prosciutto. Thread 3 pieces onto each of 8 wood skewers, alternating with cherry tomatoes. (The skewers should be soaked in water for 30 minutes beforehand to prevent burning.)

4 Brush the kabobs with a little oil and place under a hot broiler for 3–4 minutes. Turn and cook for a further 3 minutes until cooked through. Serve the kabobs with the roasted vegetables and pesto.

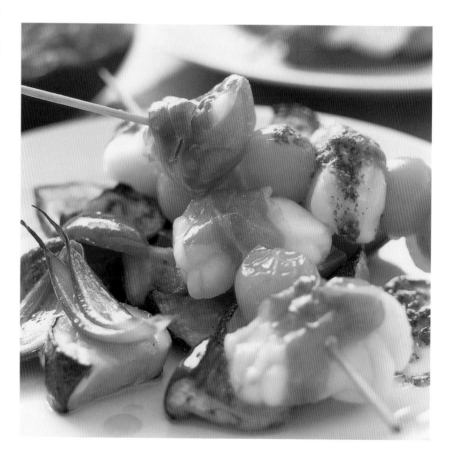

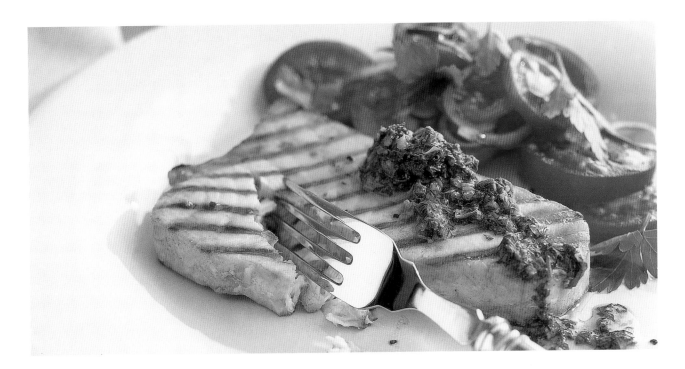

GRILLED SWORDFISH WITH SALSA VERDE

Salsa verde is a fresh, tasty sauce that works particularly well with white fish. Serve this dish with a simple tomato salad. Anchovies are a useful source of calcium, particularly for people who don't eat dairy products.

1   To make the salsa verde, place the anchovies, capers, and garlic in a food processor and blend for 30 seconds. Add the mint, basil, parsley, mustard, lemon juice, and olive oil and blend until smooth.

2   Brush a grill pan with a little olive oil and heat or heat up the barbecue. When either is hot, grill the swordfish steaks for 4–5 minutes. Turn and cook for a further 4–5 minutes. Serve with the salsa verde.

4 anchovy fillets, drained and roughly chopped

1 tablespoon (15 ml) capers, drained and rinsed

1 clove garlic, peeled

1 tablespoon (15 ml) fresh mint leaves

1 tablespoon (15 ml) fresh basil leaves

1 tablespoon (15 ml) fresh flat-leaf parsley leaves or 2 tablespoons (30 g) watercress

1 teaspoon (5 ml) Dijon mustard

Juice of 1 lemon

6 tablespoons (90 ml) olive oil, plus extra for brushing

4 swordfish steaks

Serves 4

SHRIMP & SPINACH ROULADE

This attractive roulade makes a great summer meal. Make sure the spinach is drained thoroughly before adding it to the sauce.

¼ cup (50 ml) butter, plus extra for greasing

¼ lb (125 g) frozen chopped spinach, thawed and drained

⅓ cup (75 ml) all-purpose flour

1¼ cups (300 ml) whole milk

2 eggs, separated

FOR THE FILLING

9 oz (250 g) mascarpone cheese

4 green onions, finely chopped

2 sun-dried tomatoes, finely chopped

½ lb (225 g) peeled shrimp, cooked

Salt and pepper, to taste

Serves 6

1 Grease and line a 13 × 9 in (33 × 23 cm) jelly roll pan with nonstick baking parchment. Preheat the oven to 425°F (220°C).

2 Melt the butter in a saucepan and stir in the spinach and flour. Cook for 1 minute, then add the milk. Bring to a boil, stirring continuously, then simmer for 2–3 minutes. Remove from the heat and beat in the egg yolks. In a clean bowl, stiffly whisk the egg whites, then fold into the mixture.

3 Spoon the mixture into the pan and spread out evenly with a spatula. Bake in the oven for about 15 minutes, or until well risen and firm to the touch. Turn out on to a sheet of nonstick baking parchment and peel off the lining paper. Leave covered with a damp cloth for 20 minutes to cool.

4 Meanwhile, mix together the mascarpone cheese, green onions, sun-dried tomatoes, and shrimp. Season well, then cover until the roulade is cool.

5 Spread the roulade with the shrimp filling, leaving a 1-in (2.5-cm) border. Starting at one long side, gently roll up the roulade, using the paper to help. Serve in thick slices with a crisp green salad.

PENNE WITH SHRIMP & ASPARAGUS

The lemon in this pasta enhances the flavors of the asparagus and the shrimp and makes this a light, refreshing dish.

1½ cups (375 ml) penne or other pasta

¼ lb (125 g) asparagus tips

4 tablespoons (60 ml) olive oil

3 tablespoons (45 ml) Parmesan cheese, freshly grated

Zest and juice of 1 large lemon

2 tablespoons (30 ml) fresh chives, snipped

7 oz (200 g) peeled shrimp, cooked

Serves 2

1 Cook the pasta according to the package instructions. About 4–5 minutes before it has finished cooking, add the asparagus and continue to cook until the asparagus is tender. Drain well and return to the pan.

2 Meanwhile, whisk together the olive oil, Parmesan cheese, lemon zest and juice, and chives.

3 Stir in the lemon dressing and shrimp. Cook, stirring continuously, for 4–5 minutes, or until the shrimp are hot.

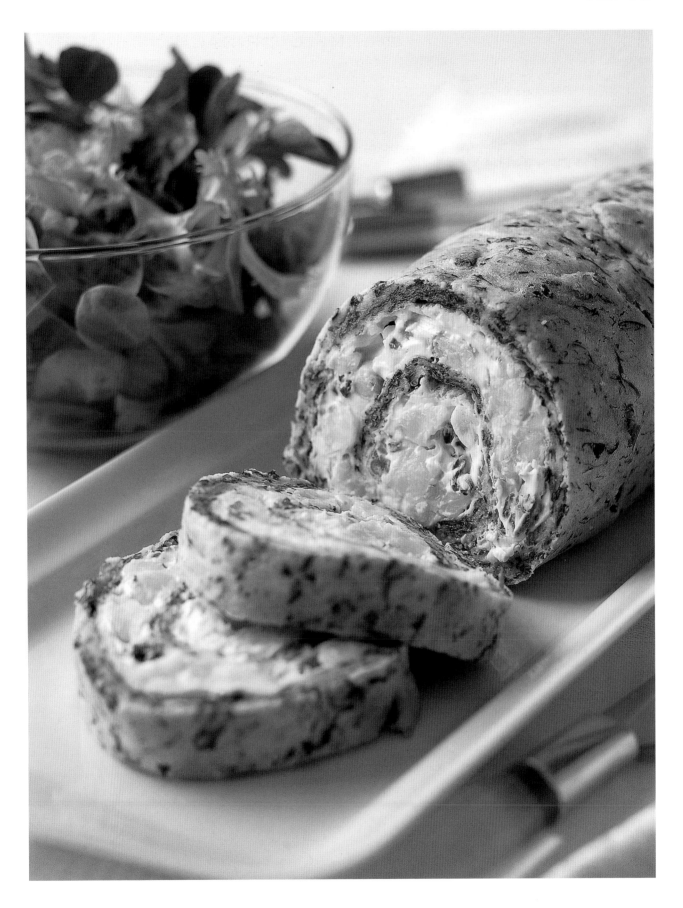

WARM LENTIL & FETA SALAD

1¼ cups (300 ml) French green lentils

1 clove garlic, peeled

1 bay leaf

4 tablespoons (60 ml) olive oil

2 tablespoons (30 ml) balsamic vinegar

1 clove garlic, crushed

½ teaspoon (2 ml) salt

½ teaspoon (2 ml) mustard powder

12 cherry tomatoes, sliced in half

3 tablespoons (45 ml) fresh parsley, chopped

2 cups (500 ml) feta cheese, crumbled

Salt and pepper, to taste

Serves 4

The subtle flavor of the lentils is perfectly complemented by the cool feta cheese, which is also a good source of calcium.

1 Place the lentils, garlic, and bay leaf in a saucepan. Cover with plenty of water and cook for 30–40 minutes, or until the lentils are just soft.

2 Whisk the olive oil, balsamic vinegar, garlic, salt, and mustard powder together in a small bowl, to make a dressing.

3 Drain the lentils and transfer to a warm serving dish. Stir in the tomatoes, parsley, and dressing. Add the feta cheese, season to taste, and serve.

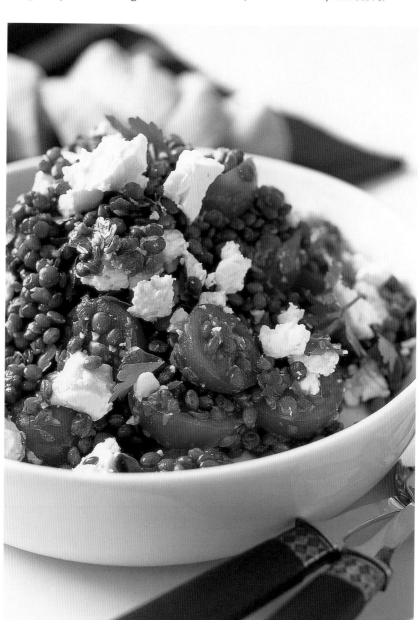

SPICED SPINACH, LENTIL, & FETA PHYLLO PIE

When working with phyllo it is essential to keep the sheets covered with a damp cloth as you work to prevent them drying out and becoming brittle.

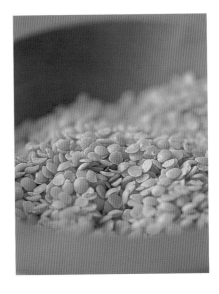

1 Preheat the oven to 375°F (190°C). Lightly grease a 9-in (22.5-cm) springform pan and set aside.

2 To make the filling, heat the oil in a saucepan. Add the onion, garlic, ground coriander, and cumin and fry gently for 10 minutes. Stir in the lentils, cover and heat through for 4–5 minutes, then mash with a fork. Transfer to a bowl and leave to cool slightly.

3 Meanwhile, cook the spinach in a large saucepan for 2–3 minutes until just wilted—there is no need to add extra water as enough clings to the leaves after washing. Refresh under cold running water. Squeeze out any excess water, shred the leaves, and add to the bowl with the spiced lentils.

4 Stir the eggs into the mixture, then add the feta, Parmesan cheese, cilantro, and season to taste. Toss to mix, then set aside.

5 Lay the phyllo pastry in the base of the prepared pan and brush with a little of the butter. Make sure the phyllo forms a solid base, but leave plenty overhanging the edges of the pan. Spoon in the filling and fold over the filo to cover the topping completely.

6 Gently scrunch the remaining sheets of phyllo and arrange on top of the pie to give a ruffled effect. Brush with the remaining butter. Bake for 30–35 minutes until golden. Allow to cool slightly before removing from the pan. Cut into wedges and serve.

---

3 tablespoons (45 ml) olive oil, plus extra for greasing

---

1 medium red onion, finely chopped

---

3 garlic cloves, crushed

---

2 teaspoons (10 ml) ground coriander

---

1 teaspoon (5 ml) ground cumin

---

2 10 oz (300 g) cans lentils, drained

---

7 cups (1.75 l) baby spinach leaves, washed

---

2 eggs, beaten

1¾ cups (425 ml) feta cheese, crumbled

---

2 tablespoons (30 ml) Parmesan cheese, freshly grated

---

4 tablespoons (60 ml) cilantro, chopped

Salt and pepper, to taste

---

12 sheets of phyllo pastry (or 6 large sheets, halved)

---

6 tablespoons (90 ml) unsalted butter, melted

Serves 6

CHEESE & LEEK SAUSAGES

These are ideal for children, but adults are sure to love them, too. They provide a good alternative to meat-filled sausages.

3¾ cups (925 ml) fine white bread crumbs

1¼ cups (300 ml) Cheddar cheese

1 small leek, trimmed and finely chopped

1 tablespoon (15 ml) fresh parsley, finely chopped

Pinch of mustard powder

Salt and pepper, to taste

1 egg, beaten

2–3 tablespoons (30–45 ml) milk

All-purpose flour, for coating

Vegetable oil, for frying or brushing

Serves 4

1 In a large bowl, mix together the bread crumbs, cheese, leek, parsley, and mustard powder. Season to taste. Add the egg and mix thoroughly, then add enough milk to bind the mixture together.

2 Divide the mixture into 8 and shape into sausages.

3 If shallow frying, roll the sausages in the flour. Heat a little oil in a large nonstick frying pan, add the sausages, and fry for about 5 minutes, or until golden brown. Alternatively, lightly brush the sausages with a little oil and cook under a hot broiler for about 3–4 minutes, turning occasionally. Serve hot or cold.

VEGETABLE PATTIES

You can use any mixed vegetables you like in these patties, such as carrots, broccoli, spinach, peas and corn. They are delicious served with a tomato salad.

¾ lb (350 g) potatoes, peeled and cut into even-sized pieces

3 tablespoons (45 ml) 2% milk

¾ lb (350 g) mixed vegetables

3 tablespoons (45 ml) vegetable oil

1 small onion, finely chopped

1 clove garlic, crushed

2 cups (500 ml) Cheddar cheese, grated

Salt and pepper, to taste

2 tablespoons (30 ml) all-purpose flour, for dusting

1 egg, beaten

2¼ cups (550 ml) fine white bread crumbs

Serves 4

1 Cook the potatoes in boiling, salted water for 15–20 minutes. Drain well, then mash with the milk. Steam the mixed vegetables and chop finely.

2 Heat 1 tablespoon (15 ml) of the oil in a large nonstick frying pan. Add the onion and garlic and cook over a medium heat for 5 minutes until soft.

3 Stir the cooked vegetables, onion and garlic mixture, and the grated cheese into the mashed potato. Season to taste, cover, and chill for 1 hour.

4 Turn the mixture onto a floured surface and shape into 8 rounds. Dip the patties into the beaten egg and coat in the bread crumbs. Chill for 15 minutes.

5 Heat the remaining oil and fry the patties, in batches, over a medium heat for 3–4 minutes on each side, or until golden brown.

BUBBLE & SQUEAK

The vegetable mixture also makes a delicious British-style "bubble and squeak." Follow the recipe up until the end of step 3. Heat 1 tablespoon (15 ml) of oil in a large nonstick frying pan, add the mixture, and fry until heated through and browned.

SPICED TOFU BURGERS

Using tofu for these vegetarian burgers ensures that they are lower in fat than those that contain a large quantity of nuts. Serve in a burger bun with mayonnaise, lettuce, and slices of tomato, not forgetting the oven fries.

1 Heat the oil in a large nonstick frying pan. Add the carrots and onion and cook, stirring continuously, for 3–4 minutes, or until the vegetables are soft. Add the ground coriander, garlic, curry paste, and tomato paste. Increase the heat and cook for 2 minutes, stirring all the time.

2 Mash the tofu with a potato masher, then stir into the vegetables along with the bread crumbs and nuts. Season well and stir until the mixture starts to stick together.

3 With floured hands, shape the mixture into 4 burgers. Heat a little of the oil in a large nonstick frying pan and fry the burgers for 3–4 minutes on each side, or until golden brown. Alternatively, to broil the burgers, brush them with a little oil and cook under a preheated broiler for about 3 minutes on each side. Drain on paper towel and serve.

1 tablespoon (15 ml) vegetable oil

1 large carrot, grated

1 large red onion, grated

2 teaspoons (10 ml) ground coriander

1 garlic clove, peeled and crushed

1 teaspoon (5 ml) hot curry paste

1 teaspoon (5 ml) sun-dried tomato paste

½ lb (225 g) tofu, drained

½ cup (125 ml) whole-wheat bread crumbs

¼ cup (50 ml) mixed nuts, toasted and finely chopped

Salt and pepper, to taste

All-purpose flour, for dusting

Vegetable oil, for frying or broiling

Makes 4 burgers

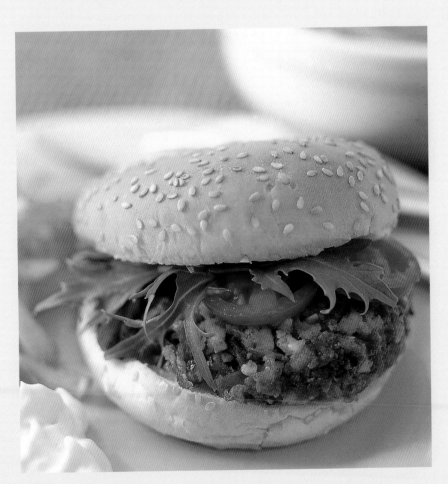

ROASTED THAI-STYLE TOFU WITH STIR-FRIED VEGETABLES

1 lb (450 g) tofu, drained

1 garlic clove, peeled and finely chopped

2 tablespoons (30 ml) hoisin sauce

2 tablespoons (30 ml) dark soy sauce

1 tablespoon (15 ml) sherry vinegar

1 tablespoon (15 ml) sweet chili sauce

1 tablespoon (15 ml) liquid honey

1 teaspoon (5 ml) sesame oil

FOR THE STIR-FRY

3 tablespoons (45 ml) sunflower oil

1 teaspoon (5 ml) sesame oil

1 medium red onion, roughly chopped

2 carrots, julienned

1 red pepper, thinly sliced

1¾ cups (425 ml) broccoli florets

1 cup (250 ml) button mushrooms, quartered

6 green onions, sliced

1 cup (250 ml) snow peas

Toasted sesame seeds, to garnish

Serves 4

Tofu is ideal for the modern healthy diet because it is low in fat and is a good source of protein. Here, the tofu is glazed in a Thai-style sauce and served with a selection of stir-fried vegetables. Egg noodles or plain boiled rice make ideal accompaniments.

1 Preheat the oven to 425°F (220°C). Cut the tofu into 1-in (2.5-cm) cubes and place in a shallow roasting pan. Mix together the garlic, hoisin sauce, soy sauce, sherry vinegar, chili sauce, honey, and sesame oil. Pour two-thirds of the marinade over the tofu and toss well, making sure the tofu is coated throughly. Roast for 25 minutes, turning once, until the tofu is deep golden brown and glazed.

2 Meanwhile, heat both oils in a wok or large nonstick frying pan. Add the red onion, carrots, red pepper, broccoli, and mushrooms and stir-fry for 3 minutes. Add the green onions and snow peas and stir-fry for a further 2 minutes.

3 Add 2 tablespoons (30 ml) of water to the remaining glaze and add this to the stir-fried vegetables. Cook for another 2–3 minutes until the vegetables are just tender, then stir in the roasted tofu. Garnish with toasted sesame seeds and serve immediately.

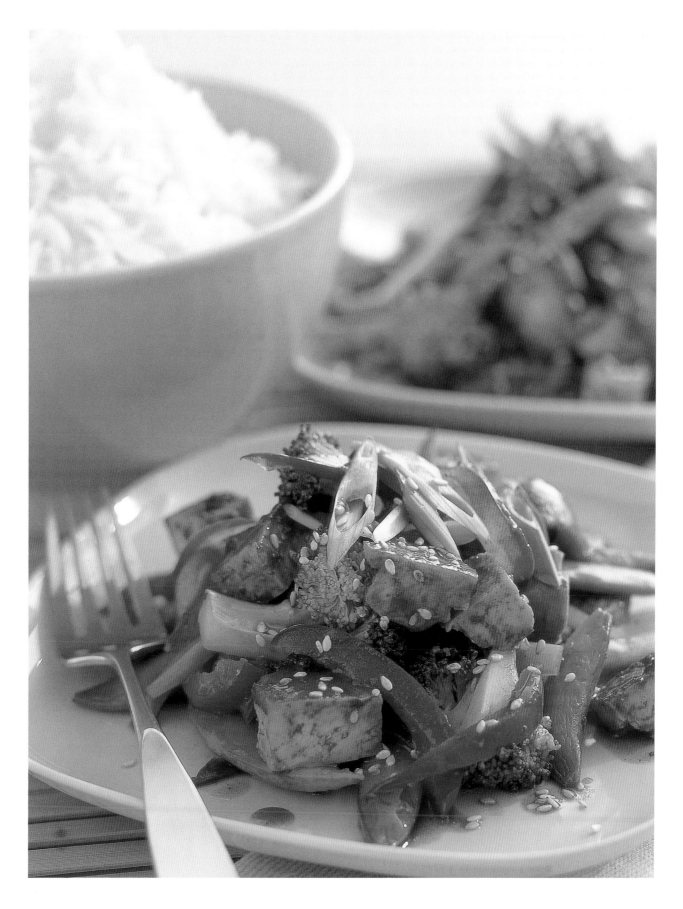

MARINATED TOFU WITH SATAY SAUCE

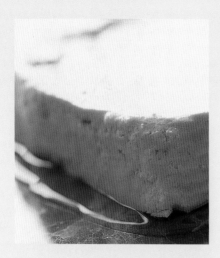

Pressed tofu is ideal for marinating because it contains less liquid and will therefore absorb more flavor. The satay sauce can be made in advance and reheated before serving.

1 Cut the tofu into ½-in (1-cm) pieces. In a shallow dish, mix together the onion, soy sauce, and sugar. Add the tofu pieces and toss, ensuring that the tofu is throughly coated. Cover and leave to marinate for at least 1 hour. Soak 8 wooden skewers in cold water for 30 minutes.

2 Meanwhile, for the satay sauce, heat the oil in a saucepan and add the garlic and chili powder. Cook, stirring, for 1–2 minutes. Add the peanut butter, sugar and lemon zest, along with 1¼ cups (300 ml) water. Bring to a simmer and cook for 4–5 minutes until the sauce thickens.

3 Heat the broiler to high. Thread the tofu onto 8 skewers. Cook for 3–4 minutes on each side, turning occasionally until browned.

4 Serve on a bed of salad greens, onions, and carrot chunks, accompanied by the satay sauce.

9 oz (250 g) pressed tofu

I small onion, finely chopped

3 tablespoons (45 ml) dark soy sauce

I teaspoon (5 ml) demerara (raw) sugar

FOR THE SATAY SAUCE

I tablespoon (15 ml) vegetable oil

I clove garlic, peeled and crushed

2 teaspoons (10 ml) chili powder

1¼ cups (300 ml) chunky peanut butter

I tablespoon (15 ml) demerara (raw) sugar

Zest of I large lemon

TO SERVE

Selection of salad greens, chopped onion, and carrot chunks

Serves 4

SATAY SAUCE WITH BROILED VEGETABLES
Broil a selection of vegetables, such as red peppers, tomatoes, zucchini, onions, or shallots and serve with the satay sauce.

HOT SPICED CHICKPEAS

This dish is delicious warm, accompanied by crusty whole-wheat bread, but can also be served cold with a wild arugula or spring mix salad.

1 Heat the oil in a large saucepan and sauté the onions for 5–7 minutes, until soft.

2 Add the turmeric and cumin seeds and fry for 1 minute, stirring frequently. Add the chickpeas, tomatoes, lemon juice, and cilantro and sauté for 4–5 minutes until heated through.

3 Season well and serve garnished with cilantro leaves and a sprinkling of cayenne pepper.

1 tablespoon (15 ml) vegetable oil

1 large red onion, roughly chopped

2 teaspoons (10 ml) ground turmeric

1 tablespoon (15 ml) cumin seeds

2 14 oz (400 g) cans chickpeas, drained and rinsed

1 lb (450 g) cherry tomatoes, halved

1 tablespoon (15 ml) lemon juice

4 tablespoons (60 ml) cilantro, chopped

Salt and pepper, to taste

Cilantro leaves, to garnish

Cayenne pepper, to garnish

Serves 6

CHICKPEA & POTATO STEW

A quick and easy stew using canned chickpeas and potatoes flavored with Indian spices. Serve with boiled pilaf rice.

1 In a large saucepan, heat the oil and cook the onion for 5 minutes until soft.

2 Add the garlic and curry paste and cook for 30 seconds, stirring frequently. Stir in the potato, chickpeas and chili and season well. Add the stock and ⅔ cup (150 ml) water. Simmer for 30 minutes.

3 Add the green onions, 3 tablespoons of chopped cilantro, lime juice, and garam masala. Reheat and simmer for 2–3 minutes. Season to taste. Garnish with the remaining chopped cilantro and serve.

CHICKPEA AND SWEET POTATO STEW
For an interesting variation on this recipe, replace the potato with sweet potato, which will give it a more mellow flavor.

2 tablespoons (30 ml) sunflower oil

2 medium red onions, chopped

4 cloves garlic, peeled and chopped

2 tablespoons (30 ml) medium-hot curry paste

1 lb (450 g) potatoes, diced

2 14 oz (400 g) cans chickpeas, drained and rinsed

1 red chili, seeded and chopped

Salt and pepper, to taste

1¼ cups (300 ml) vegetable stock

6 green onions, chopped

4 tablespoons (60 ml) cilantro, chopped

Juice of 1 lime

1 teaspoon (5 ml) garam masala

Serves 4

MIXED BEANS WITH A CORNMEAL TOPPING

Cans of navy, kidney or other beans are good to keep on hand. They are rich in soluble fiber (the type that helps reduce cholesterol levels) and are also a useful source of calcium.

FOR THE BEANS

1 tablespoon (15 ml) olive oil

1 small onion, finely chopped

2 garlic cloves, peeled and finely chopped

14 oz (400 g) can chopped tomatoes

1 cup (250 ml) vegetable stock

2 tablespoons (30 ml) dark soy sauce

3 tablespoons (45 ml) demerara (raw) sugar

1 tablespoon (15 ml) mild mustard

2 14-oz (400-g) cans of mixed beans, rinsed and drained

FOR THE TOPPING

⅓ cup (75 ml) pastry flour

⅓ cup (75 ml) cornmeal

¼ teaspoon (1 ml) salt

½ teaspoon (2 ml) baking powder

5 tablespoons (75 ml) whole milk

2 eggs, separated

1 tablespoon (15 ml) olive oil

1⅓ cups (300 ml) Cheddar cheese, grated

Serves 4

1 Heat 1 tablespoon (15 ml) of the oil in a saucepan. Add the onion and garlic and cook for 5 minutes until soft. Add the tomatoes, stock, and soy sauce. Bring to a boil, then reduce to a fast simmer and cook for about 15 minutes, or until the sauce begins to thicken.

2 Add the sugar, mustard, and mixed beans. Continue to cook for a further 5 minutes, until the beans are hot.

3 Preheat the oven to 400°C (200°C). Meanwhile, make the topping; mix the flour, cornmeal, salt, baking powder, milk, egg yolks, oil, and half of the cheese in a bowl. Beat together to make a fairly stiff batter, adding a little extra milk if necessary.

4 Beat the egg whites in a clean bowl until stiff, then, using a metal spoon, fold carefully into the batter.

5 Transfer the beans to a shallow ovenproof dish and spoon over the topping. Sprinkle over the remaining Cheddar cheese and cook for 20 minutes, until the topping is golden brown and well risen.

BUTTERNUT SQUASH & GRUYÈRE RISOTTO

You can use any type of squash or pumpkin to make this delicious creamy risotto. The secret of a good risotto is to keep it simmering slowly while you add the stock a little at a time, so it cooks evenly. Arborio rice is the best-known Italian rice and is ideal for risotto—its plump, long grains absorb liquid without losing their bite.

1. Heat the oil in a large saucepan, add the leeks, garlic, chili, rosemary, and sage and cook for 5 minutes until soft.

2. Add the rice and stir-fry for 1 minute until all the grains are glossy. Bring the vegetable stock to a steady simmer in another saucepan.

3. Add the butternut squash and stir well. Pour in ⅔ cup (150 ml) of the hot stock and stir over a medium heat until absorbed. Gradually add the remaining stock, a ladleful at a time, stirring occasionally, making sure each addition is absorbed before adding the next. Continue until the rice is tender and all the stock absorbed—this should take about 25 minutes.

4. Remove from the heat and stir in 1 cup (250 ml) of the Gruyère cheese and the cream. Cover and allow to stand for 5 minutes. Season well to taste.

5. Top with the remaining Gruyère cheese and a grinding of black pepper. Garnish with small fresh rosemary sprigs and Gruyère shavings.

4 tablespoons (60 ml) olive oil

2 leeks, trimmed and thinly sliced

2 garlic cloves, finely chopped

1 red chili, seeded and thinly sliced

1 tablespoon (15 ml) fresh rosemary, chopped

1 tablespoon (15 ml) fresh sage, chopped

1½ cups (425 ml) arborio rice

4 cups (1 liter) vegetable stock

1 lb (450 g) butternut squash, peeled, seeded, and chopped

1¼ cups (300 ml) Gruyère cheese, grated

4 tablespoons (60 ml) heavy cream

Salt and pepper, to taste

Small fresh rosemary sprigs, to garnish

Gruyère shavings, to garnish

Serves 4

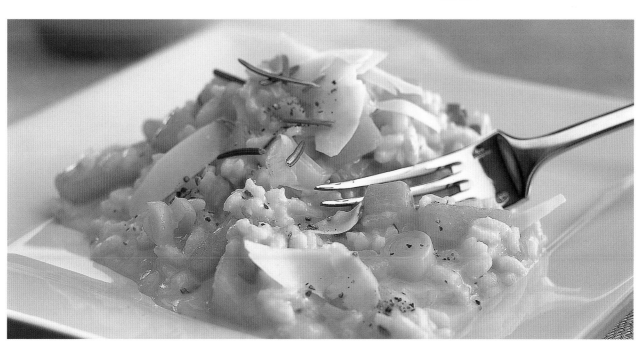

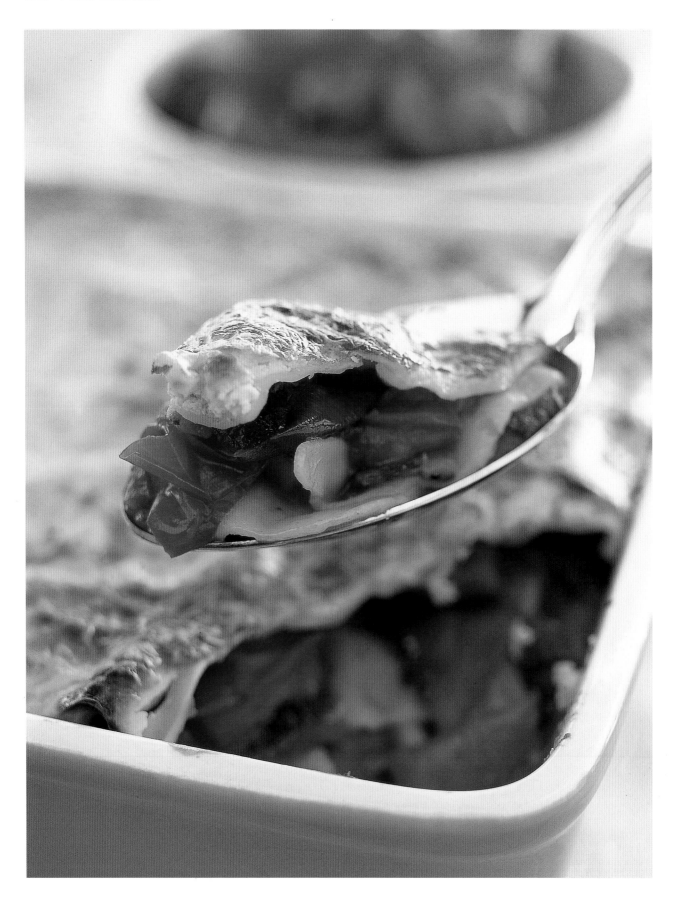

ROASTED VEGETABLE LASAGNA

Served with a tomato and basil salad, this recipe provides a healthy, balanced meal. You can use precooked lasagna, but add a little extra liquid to the vegetable and tomato mixture.

1   Preheat the oven to 375°F (190°C). Place the chopped vegetables in a large shallow roasting pan. Toss in the oil and season well. Roast for 25–30 minutes until slightly blackened. Leave to cool slightly.

2   Meanwhile, mix together the ricotta cheese with the egg, milk, and 4 tablespoons (60 ml) of the Parmesan cheese. Season well and set aside.

3   Spoon the roasted vegetables into a large bowl and mix with the canned tomatoes (use those with added garlic and herbs for extra flavor) and basil. Spoon a layer of vegetable and tomato mixture over the base of a lightly greased ovenproof dish and cover with a layer of lasagna noodles.

4   Continue with another layer of the vegetable and tomato mixture, then another layer of lasagna. Repeat this process once more, then spread the ricotta cheese mixture evenly over the top and sprinkle with the remaining Parmesan cheese. Bake for 30 minutes or until golden brown and bubbling.

5   Leave the lasagna to stand for 5 minutes before serving.

1 large zucchini, roughly chopped

1 red pepper, seeded and chopped

1 red onion, roughly chopped

1 small eggplant, chopped

2 tablespoons (30 ml) olive oil

Salt and pepper, to taste

9 oz (250 g) ricotta cheese

1 egg

4 tablespoons (60 ml) whole milk

6 tablespoons (90 ml) Parmesan cheese, grated

28 oz (800 g) canned chopped tomatoes

2 tablespoons (30 ml) fresh basil, chopped

8–10 fresh lasagna noodles

Serves 4

PAPPARDELLE WITH SPICY TOMATO SAUCE & RICOTTA

Ricotta cheese is surprisingly low in fat compared with many other cheeses, but still provides useful amounts of calcium. The creaminess of the ricotta perfectly balances the heat of the sauce. If time is short, use ready-made arrabbiata sauce instead of making your own tomato sauce.

1   Heat the oil in large saucepan, add the onion, garlic, ground coriander and cumin and cook for 5 minutes, or until the onions are soft. Add the tomatoes, tomato paste, red wine, and seasoning, bring to a boil, then simmer for about 30 minutes, or until the sauce has reduced by about half.

2   Cook the pasta according to the package instructions and drain well.

3   Transfer the pasta to a serving dish, add the tomato sauce, then stir in the ricotta cheese. Garnish with fresh basil and serve immediately.

1 tablespoon (15 ml) olive oil

1 large red onion, finely chopped

1 clove garlic, peeled and finely chopped

1 teaspoon (5 ml) ground coriander

1 teaspoon (5 ml) ground cumin

28 oz (800 g) canned chopped tomatoes

1 tablespoon (15 ml) tomato paste

⅔ cup (150 ml) red wine

Salt and pepper, to taste

2¼ cups (550 ml) pappardelle, or other pasta

7 oz (200 g) ricotta cheese

Fresh basil, chopped, to garnish

Serves 4

BROCCOLI & GRUYÈRE SOUFFLÉ

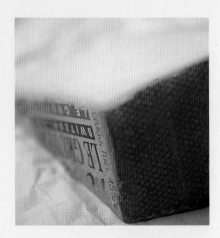

Broccoli is good source of vitamin K, which is an important nutrient for bone health. It also provides useful amounts of calcium, so is particularly good for people on a dairy-free diet.

1 Preheat the oven to 350°F (180°C). Grease 6 ramekin dishes and place on a baking tray. Steam the broccoli over a pan of boiling water for 8 minutes until tender.

2 Melt the butter in a saucepan, stir in the flour and cook for 1 minute. Gradually stir in the milk and bring to a boil. Cook, stirring continuously, until the mixture has thickened.

3 Pour the sauce into a food processor, add the broccoli, and purée until the mixture is smooth.

4 Transfer the mixture to a bowl, allow to cool slightly, then stir in the egg yolks and Gruyère cheese. Season to taste.

5 In a clean bowl, whisk the egg whites until stiff, then lightly fold into the sauce mixture.

6 Spoon into the ramekin dishes, transfer to the oven, and cook for 20–25 minutes, or until the soufflés are just firm to the touch. Serve immediately.

Butter, for greasing

½ lb (225 g) broccoli florets

3 tablespoons (45 ml) butter

3 tablespoons (45 ml) all-purpose flour

1 cup (250 ml) whole milk

3 eggs, separated

1¼ cups (300 ml) Gruyère cheese, grated

Salt and pepper, to taste

Serves 6

SPINACH AND GRUYÈRE SOUFFLÉ
Replace the broccoli with 8 oz (225 g) cooked spinach. Squeeze any excess moisture from the spinach and follow the instructions above.

Mediterranean Stuffed Peppers with Couscous

Couscous is an ideal accompaniment to these tasty and healthy stuffed red peppers. They can also be served on top of toasted ciabatta rubbed with garlic, accompanied by an arugula or spring mix salad.

1 Preheat the oven to 350°F (180°C). Cut the peppers in half through the stalks. Scoop out the seeds and the white ribs, leaving the stalk intact. Put the pepper halves cut-side up into a large roasting pan and set aside.

2 To remove the tomato skins, mark a cross in the top of each one and put them into a bowl. Cover with boiling water and leave for 1 minute, then drain. Leave to cool slightly then peel off the skin and cut the tomatoes into wedges.

3 Mix the tomato wedges, garlic, capers, olives, and oregano leaves together, then spoon into the pepper halves. Drizzle with the olive oil and season well.

4 Roast for 35 minutes. Remove from the oven and sprinkle with feta and pine nuts or almonds. Return to the oven and cook for a further 10 minutes, or until the feta has melted and the nuts are lightly golden.

5 Meanwhile, put the couscous into a large bowl and add the boiling water or vegetable stock. Leave for about 5 minutes until the stock is absorbed and the couscous soft. Chop the parsley, reserving several sprigs to garnish. Fluff up the couscous mixture with a fork and toss in the parsley, green onions, lemon zest, and a drizzle of olive oil.

6 To serve, place a little couscous and 2 roasted pepper halves onto each of 4 serving plates. Garnish with parsley and a grinding of black pepper.

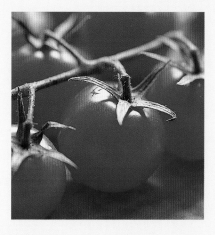

FOR THE STUFFED PEPPERS

4 large red peppers

12 cherry tomatoes, halved

3 cloves garlic, peeled and thinly sliced

1 teaspoon (5 ml) capers, drained and rinsed

8 pitted black olives, roughly chopped

1 tablespoon (15 ml) fresh oregano leaves

4 tablespoons (60 ml) virgin olive oil

Salt and pepper, to taste

1⅓ cups (325 ml) feta cheese, crumbled

2 tablespoons (30 ml) pine nuts or slivered almonds

FOR THE COUSCOUS

1 cup (250 ml) couscous

1¼ cups (300 ml) boiling water or hot vegetable stock

2 tablespoons (30 ml) fresh flat-leaf parsley, plus extra to garnish

4 green onions, shredded

Zest of 1 lemon

Olive oil, for drizzling

Serves 4

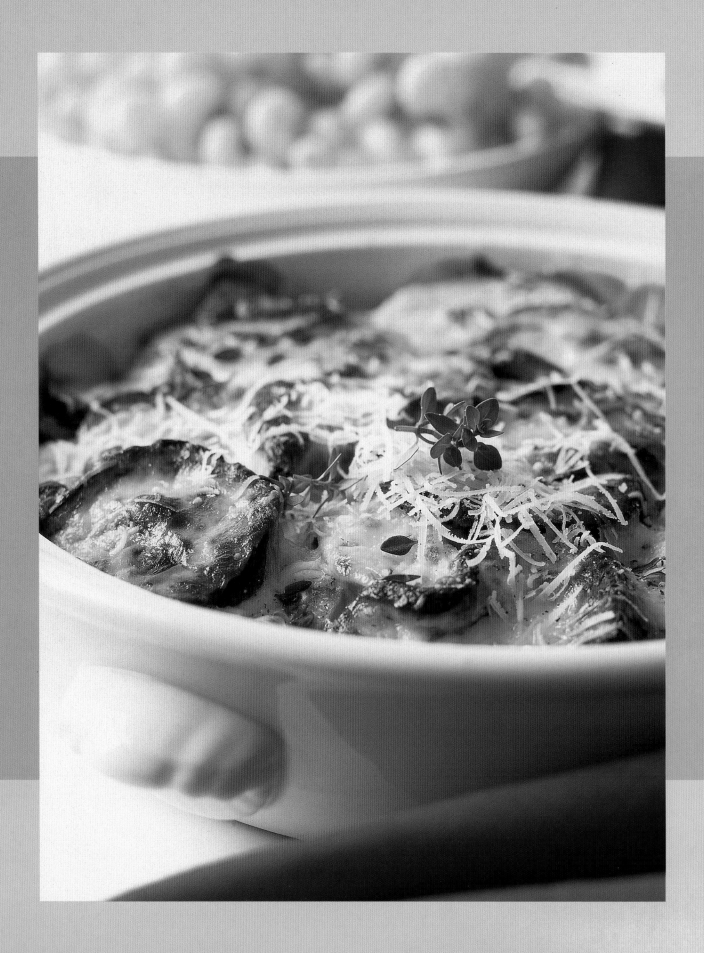

5 On the Side

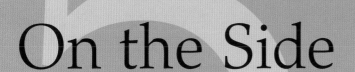

Accompaniments can sometimes become a second thought when preparing a meal, so this chapter offers creative ideas for vegetable side dishes and salads that will boost the flavor and nutritional value of any dish.

GREEN BEANS WITH FETA & SUN-DRIED TOMATOES

The combination of feta and sun-dried tomatoes gives this accompaniment a classic Mediterranean flavor. It works well with plain broiled meat or fish.

9 oz (250 g) green beans, trimmed

¾ cup (175 ml) feta cheese, crumbled

½ cup (125 ml) sun-dried tomatoes in oil, sliced into thin strips

Salt and pepper, to taste

Serves 4

1 Cook the beans in a large pan of boiling salted water for 3–4 minutes or until just tender. Drain well.

2 Toss the beans with the feta cheese and sun-dried tomatoes. Season to taste and serve.

ROASTED BABY CARROTS WITH PARMESAN & CILANTRO TOPPING

The Parmesan cheese and cilantro topping is quick and tasty and works well with most vegetables. Adding a cheesy crust is also a great way to persuade kids to eat vegetables.

1⅓ lb (600 g) baby carrots

1 tablespoon (15 ml) sunflower oil

1 tablespoon (15 ml) unsalted butter

Salt and pepper, to taste

3 tablespoons (45 ml) cilantro, chopped

½ cup (125 ml) Parmesan cheese, freshly grated

Serves 4

1 Preheat the oven to 400°F (200°C). Put the carrots in a large saucepan of boiling water and boil for 3 minutes. Drain well.

2 Place the carrots in a shallow ovenproof dish with the oil, butter, and seasoning. Roast in the oven for 15 minutes.

3 Meanwhile, mix the cilantro and Parmesan cheese together in a small bowl. Remove the carrots from the oven and sprinkle with the mixture. Return to the oven for another 10 minutes, until the carrots are tender and lightly golden.

SPICY ROAST BABY CARROTS WITH FETA

Follow steps 1 and 2 as above. With a pestle and mortar, grind together 1 teaspoon (5 ml) coriander seeds, 1 teaspoon (5 ml) ground cardamom, 1 bay leaf, 1 teaspoon (5 ml) cumin seeds, 6 peppercorns, 1 teaspoon (5 ml) hot paprika and half a cinnamon stick. Sprinkle this mixture over the carrots and toss lightly, then crumble 2 cups (500 ml) feta cheese over it. Return the carrots to the oven for 10 minutes until they are tender and the cheese has melted.

ASIAN-STYLE BROCCOLI

Lightly steamed broccoli is a useful source of calcium. It also provides good amounts of beta carotene, vitamin C, vitamin B₆, folic acid and niacin.

1 Cook the broccoli in a large pan of boiling salted water for 1–2 minutes. Immediately plunge the broccoli into ice-cold water to stop it from cooking further. Drain well and blot dry with absorbent kitchen paper.

2 Heat the sesame and sunflower oils in a wok or large frying pan. Add the garlic, chili, and ginger and stir-fry for 2–3 minutes. Add the broccoli and soy sauce and continue to cook for 1 minute. Sprinkle with the sesame seeds and serve.

1lb (450 g) broccoli, divided into small florets

2 teaspoons (10 ml) sesame oil

2 teaspoons (10 ml) sunflower oil

1 clove garlic, peeled and finely chopped

1 red chili, seeded and finely chopped

½ in (1 cm) fresh ginger, chopped

1 tablespoon (15 ml) light soy sauce

1 teaspoon (5 ml) sesame seeds

Serves 4

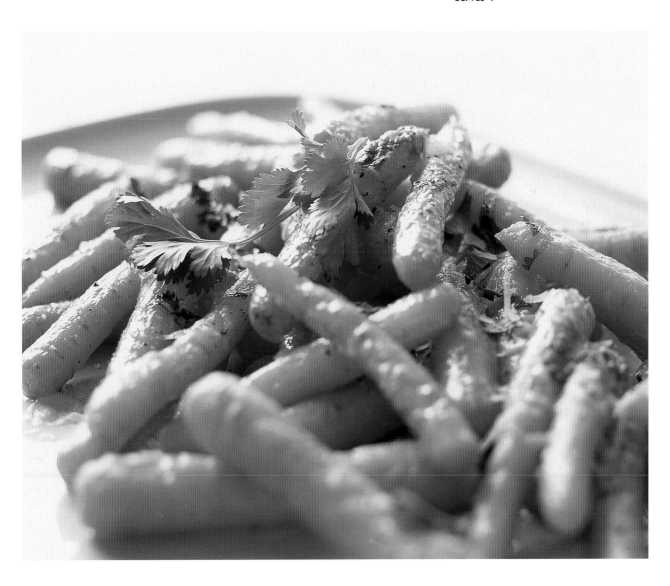

HONEYED PARSNIPS WITH SESAME SEEDS

1½ lbs (700 g) parsnips, peeled

¼ cup (50 ml) butter

2 tablespoons (30 ml) honey

2 tablespoons (30 ml) sesame seeds, toasted

Salt and pepper, to taste

Fresh thyme sprigs, to garnish

Serves 4

Sesame seeds are a good source of calcium, particularly for anyone following a dairy-free diet. One tablespoon of sesame seeds will provide around 10 percent of the daily calcium requirement for women aged between 19 and 50. It also provides around 10 percent of the daily iron requirement and 17 percent of the daily vitamin B_6 requirement.

1 Cut the parsnips in half lengthwise and in half again. (If using older, tougher parsnips, cut into quarters and remove the woody cores.) Add the parsnips to a pan of boiling salted water and cook for 5 minutes.

2 Meanwhile, melt the butter in a large saucepan. Add the honey and heat gently, stirring until it is dissolved.

3 Drain the parsnips, then add the honey mixture to the pan and toss well to coat the parsnips. Cook over a moderate heat for about 10 minutes, shaking the pan frequently, until the parsnips are golden brown. Sprinkle with the sesame seeds and toss through. Season to taste.

4 Transfer to a warmed serving dish and garnish with thyme sprigs.

PARSNIPS WITH A SWEET LIME GLAZE
Prepare the parsnips as in step 1. Remove the zest from 1 lime and reserve. Put the juice of the lime, ¼ cup (50 ml) butter and 3 tablespoons (45 ml) soft light brown sugar in a large pan and heat until the butter is melted and the sugar dissolved. Follow the recipe as above, using the sweet lime butter instead of the honey mixture. After cooking, stir in ¾ cup (175 ml) walnuts instead of the sesame seeds. Garnish with the lime zest and fresh thyme sprigs.
This sweet lime glaze can be used with any sweet root vegetables, such as sweet potatoes or carrots.

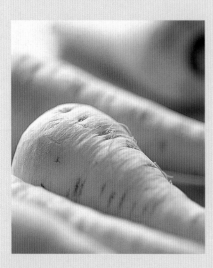

FANTAIL ROAST POTATOES WITH SESAME SEEDS

A roast wouldn't be the same without roast potatoes, and these look attractive as well as tasting great. The sesame seeds give them a crunchy, slightly nutty taste and boost the calcium content of the dish. They are also an ideal source of potassium, which is an important ingredient for healthy bones.

1 Preheat the oven to 350°F (180°C). Place the potatoes in a large saucepan, cover with salted cold water, and bring to a boil, then cook for 3 minutes. Drain well and rinse under cold running water to cool slightly.

2 Using a sharp knife, slice into each potato at ⅛–¼ in (3–5 mm) intervals, cutting three-quarters of the way through.

3 Heat a thin layer of oil in a large roasting pan in the oven. Add the potatoes and turn them in the oil to coat. Place cut-side up and sprinkle with the sesame seeds.

4 Roast the potatoes for about 1–1¼ hours, basting occasionally. Increase the oven temperature to 425°F (220°C) and roast for a further 15 minutes, until the outside of the potatoes is crisp and golden brown. Serve garnished with parsley sprigs.

4 lb (1.8 kg) potatoes, peeled and cut into large even-sized pieces

Salt and pepper, to taste

Vegetable oil, for basting

2 tablespoons (30 ml) sesame seeds

Fresh parsley sprigs, to garnish

Serves 6

RED PESTO FANTAIL ROAST POTATOES

Follow the main recipe as above, omitting the sesame seeds. After the potatoes have been roasting for 1–1¼ hours, remove from the oven. Carefully pull the potatoes apart and spread a little red pesto between each slice—use about 3 tablespoons (45 ml) of pesto altogether. Close the potatoes back up and baste the tops with a little oil from the roasting pan. Increase the oven temperature, as in the main recipe, and roast for a further 15 minutes. Serve with a salad of arugula, crumbled feta, cherry tomatoes, marinated red pepper, and a drizzle of olive oil.

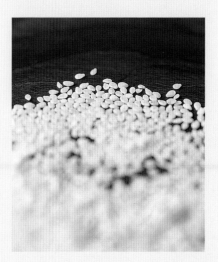

SWEET POTATO & ANCHOVY GRATIN

1¾ cups (450 ml) whole milk

⅔ cup (150 ml) heavy cream

Butter, for greasing

2¼ lbs (1 kg) sweet potatoes, sliced

2 red onions, sliced

2 oz (50 g) canned anchovies, drained and cut in half lengthways

2 cloves garlic, peeled and finely chopped

Salt and pepper, to taste

1¼ cups (300 ml) Gruyère cheese, grated

Serves 6

Sweet potatoes are an excellent source of beta carotene and provide good amounts of vitamin C and potassium, which are important for bone health. This dish is a perfect accompaniment for roast lamb.

1   Put the milk and cream into a saucepan. Bring slowly to a boil, remove from the heat, and set aside.

2   Preheat the oven to 400°F (200°C). Grease a 3-pint (1.8-l) ovenproof dish.

3   Layer the potatoes and onions in the dish with the anchovies, garlic, and seasoning between the layers.

4   Pour the warm milk and cream over the potato and onion mixture. Cover the dish with foil, place on a baking pan and bake for 1 hour. Remove the foil and sprinkle with the Gruyère cheese. Bake for a further 15–20 minutes until tender and golden. Serve hot.

EGGPLANT & TOMATO GRATIN

9 oz (250 g) mascarpone cheese

4 tablespoons (60 ml) Parmesan cheese, freshly grated

Salt and pepper, to taste

2 medium eggplants

Light olive oil or vegetable oil, for frying

6 plum tomatoes, sliced

2 cloves garlic, peeled and roughly chopped

2 eggs, beaten

Fresh thyme leaves, to garnish

Serves 6

This creamy vegetable gratin is an excellent accompaniment to lamb. It also makes a tasty vegetarian main course when served with pasta.

1   Preheat the oven to 400°F (200°C). In a saucepan, heat the mascarpone cheese for 1–2 minutes until smooth. Stir in half the Parmesan cheese and season well. Set aside.

2   Thinly slice the eggplants. Pour enough oil into a large nonstick frying pan to cover the base. Heat until the oil is very hot, then add a layer of eggplant slices—you will need to cook the eggplant in 2 batches. Fry over a moderate heat until golden brown on both sides, turning once. Remove with a slotted spoon and drain on paper towel. Repeat with the remaining eggplant slices, adding more oil, if necessary.

3   Arrange alternate layers of eggplant and tomato in a greased ovenproof dish. Sprinkle a little garlic, a little salt, and plenty of pepper in between each layer.

4   Beat the eggs into the cheese sauce, then slowly pour over the eggplant and tomato. Sprinkle the remaining cheese over the top. Bake for 20 minutes, or until the topping is golden and bubbling. Garnish with thyme leaves and serve hot.

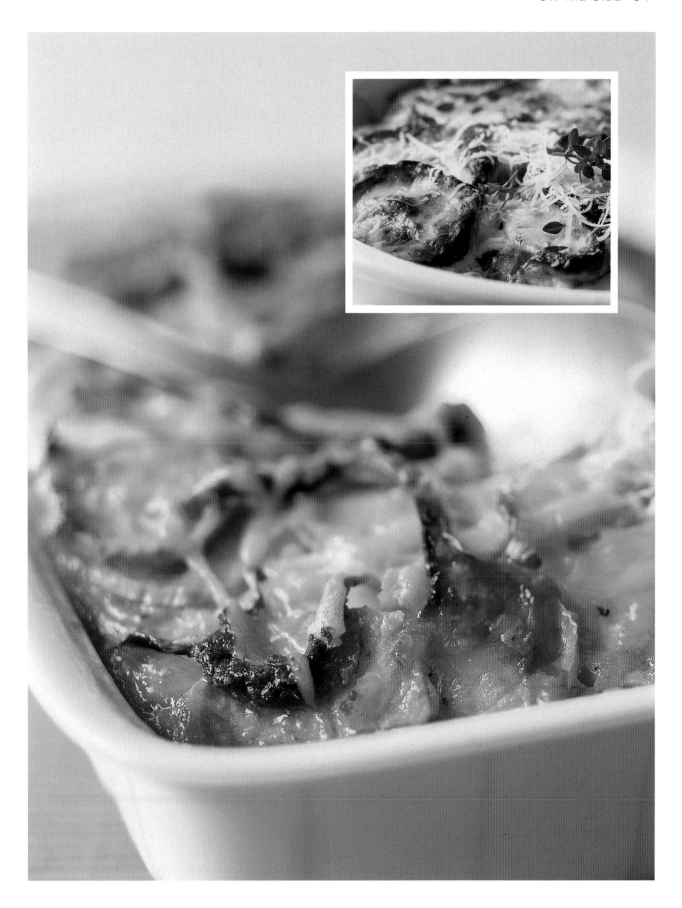

CAULIFLOWER & BROCCOLI CHEESE

Adding a rich, creamy mascarpone sauce to a combination of vegetables transforms this family favorite.

¾ lb (350 g) cauliflower florets

¾ lb (350 g) broccoli florets

1 teaspoon (5 ml) vegetable oil

4 green onions, finely shredded

1 lb (500 g) mascarpone cheese

1¼ cups (300 ml) Cheddar cheese, grated

Salt and pepper, to taste

3 tablespoons (45 ml) fresh whole-wheat bread crumbs

Fresh flat-leaf parsley, roughly chopped, to garnish

Serves 6

1　Preheat the oven to 400°F (200°C). Put the cauliflower and broccoli in a pan of boiling salted water. Bring back to a boil and cook for 6–7 minutes until just tender, then drain thoroughly. Place in an ovenproof dish.

2　Heat the oil in a frying pan and stir-fry the green onions for 2–3 minutes, until softened. Add the mascarpone cheese and cook for 1–2 minutes until smooth. Stir in half of the Cheddar cheese and season well.

3　Pour the cheese sauce evenly over the cauliflower and broccoli. Sprinkle with the bread crumbs and the remaining cheese and bake for 25 minutes, until the topping is golden and bubbling. Garnish with flat-leaf parsley and a grinding of fresh black pepper.

APPLE, WALNUT & WATERCRESS SALAD

Apples and walnuts are a classic combination and help to give this salad a wonderful crunchy texture. Watercress provides a useful source of calcium, particularly for people on dairy-free diets.

½ cup (125 ml) walnut halves

2 teaspoons (10 ml) sherry vinegar

3 tablespoons (45 ml) olive oil

1 tablespoon (15 ml) walnut oil

Salt and pepper, to taste

1 small red onion, peeled and thinly sliced

2 crisp green eating apples, quartered, cored and sliced

1 cup (250 ml) watercress

Serves 4

1　To make the salad dressing, chop half the walnuts very finely by hand, or in a food processor. Place in a bowl and whisk in the vinegar, olive oil, and walnut oil and season with salt and pepper. Set aside until ready to use.

2　Toss the onion, apple, and watercress together in a bowl. Whisk the salad dressing and drizzle it over the salad. Sprinkle with the remaining walnut halves to serve.

POTATO SALAD WITH BLUE CHEESE DRESSING

A high-calcium version of a popular side dish, this is perfect as an accompaniment, and also great for a picnic or buffet lunch.

1 Place the potatoes in a pan of boiling salted water and boil for 15–20 minutes, until cooked through.

2 Whisk together the fromage frais and milk, then stir in the cheese.

3 Drain the potatoes well and place in a serving dish. Cover with the blue cheese dressing and sprinkle with chives. Stir well to ensure the potatoes are coated with the dressing, then serve.

1¼ lbs (550 g) new potatoes, sliced in half

5 tablespoons (60 ml) sour cream or yogurt

3 tablespoons (45 ml) 2% milk

1¼ cups (300 ml) Stilton or other blue cheese, crumbled or chopped into small pieces

2 tablespoons (30 ml) fresh chives, chopped

Serves 4

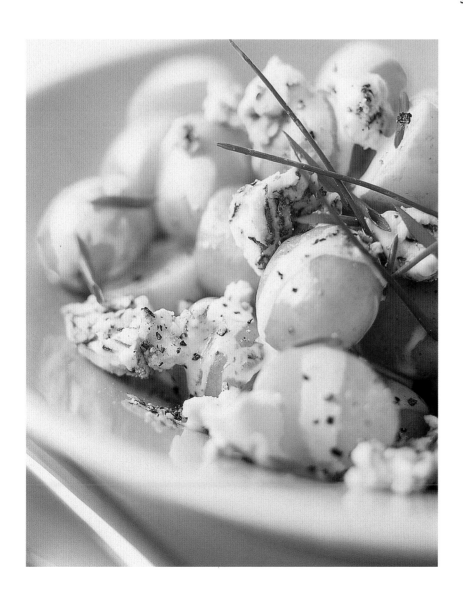

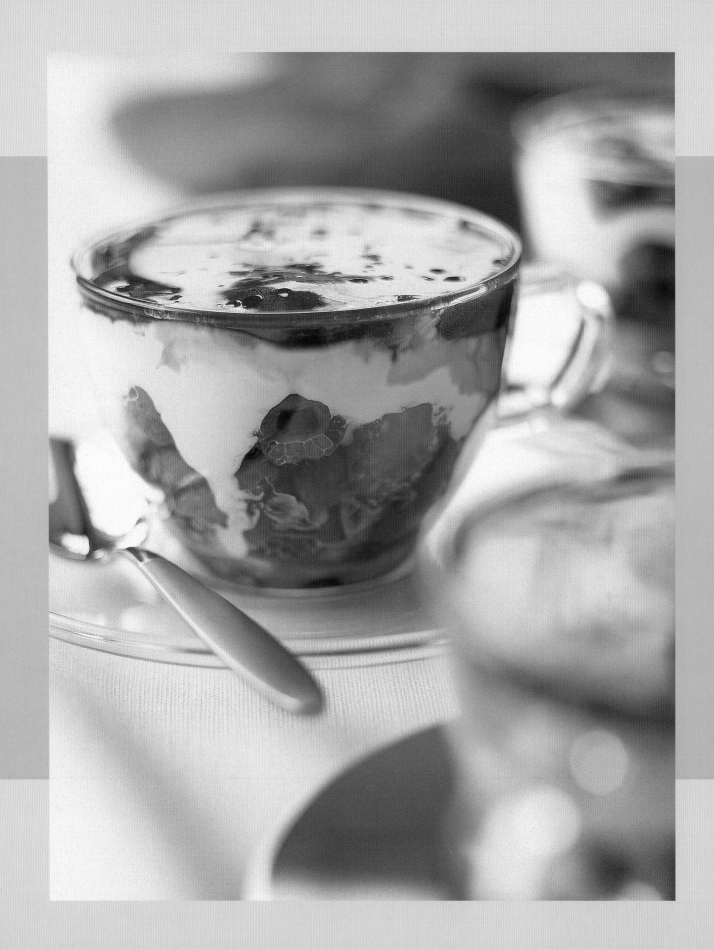

6 Desserts & Treats

THOUGH WE DON'T NORMALLY
THINK OF DESSERTS AS BEING
NUTRITIOUS, THEY CAN PROVIDE
GOOD QUANTITIES OF VITAMINS
AND MINERALS. THE RECIPES THAT
FOLLOW INCORPORATE CAREFULLY
CHOSEN, HEALTHY INGREDIENTS,
AND ALL TASTE DELICIOUS.

FUDGY NUT PIE

½ lb (225 g) ready-made shortcrust pastry or prepared pie shell

Flour, for dusting

3 oz (75 g) dark chocolate, broken into small pieces

¼ cup (50 ml) butter

1¼ cup (300 ml) dark brown sugar

½ cup (125 ml) soft light brown sugar

⅜ cup (100 ml) whole milk

⅓ cup (75 ml) corn syrup

1 teaspoon (5 ml) vanilla extract

½ teaspoon (2 ml) salt

3 eggs

1 cup (250 ml) mixed nuts, chopped

Confectioners' sugar, for dusting

Serves 6

This dessert is deliciously indulgent and is bound to be a hit with the whole family. Serve with vanilla ice cream or crème fraîche.

1 Roll out the pastry on a lightly floured surface and use to line a 9-in (23-cm) loose-bottomed, 1½-in (4-cm) deep, flan tin. Place on a baking pan, cover, and chill for 30 minutes. Preheat the oven to 400°F (200°C).

2 Prick the pastry with a fork, then line with a large sheet of parchment or foil paper and fill with dried beans. Bake for 10–15 minutes, then carefully remove the paper and the beans and return to the oven for a further 5 minutes, until the base is firm to the touch and lightly golden. Remove from the oven and set aside while making the filling.

3 To make the filling, melt the chocolate and butter in a large bowl over hot water. Remove from the heat and add the sugar, milk, corn syrup, vanilla extract, salt, and eggs. Beat with a wooden spoon until smooth, then stir in the nuts.

4 Pour the filling into the pastry shell and bake at 350°F (180°C) for 45–55 minutes, until puffy and golden. Leave to cool. Dust with confectioners' sugar to serve.

SPICED APPLE & RAISIN CRÊPES

FOR THE FILLING

½ cup (125 ml) raisins

3 tablespoons (45 ml) dark rum

2 lbs (900 g) crisp green eating apples, peeled, cored and sliced

5 tablespoons (75 ml) water

3–4 tablespoons (45–60 ml) superfine sugar

Pinch of ground cinnamon

A sweet treat that isn't loaded with fat or calories, these crêpes are delicious served on their own, or with a scoop of vanilla ice cream.

1 To make the filling, place the raisins in a small bowl, cover with the rum, and leave to stand for 30 minutes. Place the apples and water in a large pan, cover, and cook gently for about 10 minutes, stirring occasionally. Stir in the sugar, cinnamon and soaked raisins.

2 To make the crêpes, place the flour and salt in a large bowl. Add the egg and half the milk and mix for 1 minute until the mixture is bubbly—use an electric hand mixer if you have one. Stir in the rest of the milk. Pour the batter into a jug and leave to stand for 20 minutes. Add more milk as needed to obtain the consistency of very thick cream.

3 Heat a 7-in (18-cm) crêpe pan or heavy-bottomed frying pan. Add a little oil and, when it starts to smoke, pour in just enough batter to thinly coat the base of the pan. Cook over a moderate heat for about 1 minute or until the bottom is golden brown. Turn the crêpe over and cook on the other side for another 30 seconds. Slide the crêpe onto a plate, cover with foil, and keep warm in a low oven 300°F (150°C) while you make the rest of the crêpes. Add extra oil to the pan as necessary.

4 Gently reheat the apple mixture. Spoon a little of the mixture into the middle of each crêpe and roll. Serve with plain yogurt.

FOR THE CRÊPES

I cup (250 ml) sifted all-purpose flour

Pinch of salt

I extra large egg

1¼ cups (300 ml) 2% milk

Sunflower oil, for frying

Plain yogurt, to serve

Serves 4 (makes 8 crêpes)

RICH CHOCOLATE & FIG PUDDINGS WITH CHOCOLATE SAUCE

The chocolate and figs complement each other perfectly to produce these wonderfully rich, fruity desserts. A generous spoonful of crème fraîche or whipped cream is a good accompaniment.

1 Preheat the oven to 350°F (180°C). Mix the figs and syrup together and divide the mixture into 6 buttered ¼ pint (150 ml) dariole (baba) molds or ramekins.

2 Cream the butter and sugar together until light and fluffy, then beat in the eggs, a little at a time. Sift the flour, baking powder, and cocoa powder together and fold into the egg mixture. Stir in the melted chocolate and bread crumbs.

3 Spoon the mixture into the molds until they are two-thirds full. Cover with foil and place in a roasting pan containing enough hot water to come halfway up the molds. Bake for 35–40 minutes, then leave to stand for 5 minutes.

4 Meanwhile, make the chocolate sauce. Place the chocolate and butter in a bowl over a saucepan of hot water and stir until melted. Add the milk and rum and stir for 1 minute.

5 Turn out the cake and sprinkle with chocolate shavings. Serve with the chocolate sauce poured on top.

¾ cup (175 ml) chopped dried figs

4 tablespoons (60 ml) maple syrup

½ cup (125 ml) soft unsalted butter, plus extra for greasing

⅔ cup (150 ml) packed light brown sugar

3 eggs, lightly beaten

½ cup (125 ml) self-rising flour

I teaspoon (5 ml) baking powder

I tablespoon (15 ml) cocoa powder

4 oz (110 g) chocolate (with at least 70% cocoa solid), melted

1½ cups (375 ml) fresh white bread crumbs

Chocolate shavings, for sprinkling

FOR THE CHOCOLATE SAUCE

4 oz (110 g) dark chocolate

2 tablespoons (30 ml) butter

I tablespoon (15 ml) whole milk

I tablespoon (15 ml) rum

Serves 6

Dates Stuffed with Ricotta

½ cup (125 ml) ricotta cheese

1 tablespoon (15 ml) confectioners' sugar

6 fresh dates

2 tablespoons (30 ml) pistachio nuts, chopped

Serves 2

This sweet treat makes a light dessert that is perfect for after a heavy meal. The cool, creamy ricotta cheese provides a delicious complement to the sweetness of the dates.

1 Mix the ricotta and sugar together in a small bowl.

2 Make a lengthwise cut in each date and remove the pit.

3 Spoon a little of the ricotta mixture into the center of each date. Sprinkle with a few chopped pistachio nuts and serve.

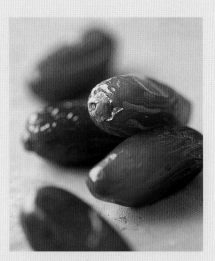

Brandied Prunes with Yogurt

2 cups (500 ml) pitted dried prunes

½ cup (125 ml) large seedless Thompson raisins

⅔ cup (150 ml) cold unsweetened tea

3 tablespoons (45 ml) brandy

½ cup (125 ml) plain or vanilla-flavored yogurt

2 tablespoons (30 ml) confectioners' sugar

6 brandy or ginger snaps, to serve

Serves 6

Plump and succulent prunes make a light and tasty dessert. Prunes are a good source of fiber and provide useful amounts of calcium and iron.

1 Place the prunes and raisins in a large bowl and cover with the tea and brandy. Cover and leave to soak for at least 6 hours, or preferably overnight.

2 When ready to serve, beat together the yogurt and confectioners' sugar. Spoon the brandied prunes into serving bowls and top each with a spoonful of the yogurt mixture and a brandy snap.

LEMON & STRAWBERRY CHEESECAKE

This fresh, lemony cheesecake makes a perfect dinner party dessert or a snack with morning coffee.

1. To make the base, place the cookies in a plastic bag, seal, then crush with a rolling pin to make fine crumbs. Melt the butter in a saucepan, then stir in the cookie crumbs and raw sugar. Press the mixture into the base and sides of an 8 x 2 in (20 x 5.8 cm) springform pan and chill until set.

2. To make the filling, place the lemon zest in a bowl. Add the cream cheese and condensed milk and beat until smooth. Very gradually beat in the lemon juice until the mixture is thick and creamy. In another bowl, whip the cream until it forms soft peaks, then fold into the cream cheese mixture.

3. Spoon the cheesecake mixture onto the cookie base and swirl the top with the back of a spoon. Arrange the strawberries cut-side down around the edge and chill for 1 hour.

4. For the strawberry sauce, put half the strawberries into a bowl and stir in the sugar and orange liqueur. Chill for 1 hour, then blend in a food processor or blender until smooth. Pass the purée through a fine nylon sieve to remove the seeds, then stir in the remaining strawberries and the orange zest.

5. To serve, remove the cheesecake from the pan and slice. Decorate with mint sprigs and serve with the strawberry sauce.

LEMON & RASPBERRY CHEESECAKE
Replace the strawberries with raspberries in both the filling and the sauce.

FOR THE CHEESECAKE BASE

4¾ cups (1.2 l) graham crackers

½ cup (125 ml) butter

1 tablespoon (15 ml) demerara (raw) sugar

FOR THE FILLING

Zest of 1 lemon

8 oz (225 g) cream cheese

¾ cup (175 ml) canned sweetened condensed milk

Juice of 3 lemons

¾ cup (175 ml) heavy cream

¼ lb (125 g) fresh strawberries, halved

FOR THE STRAWBERRY SAUCE

1 lb (450 g) small strawberries, cut into quarters

¼ cup (50 ml) superfine sugar

2 tablespoons (30 ml) orange liqueur

Zest of 1 orange

Fresh mint sprigs, to decorate

Serves 6–8

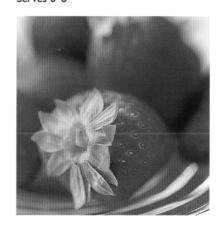

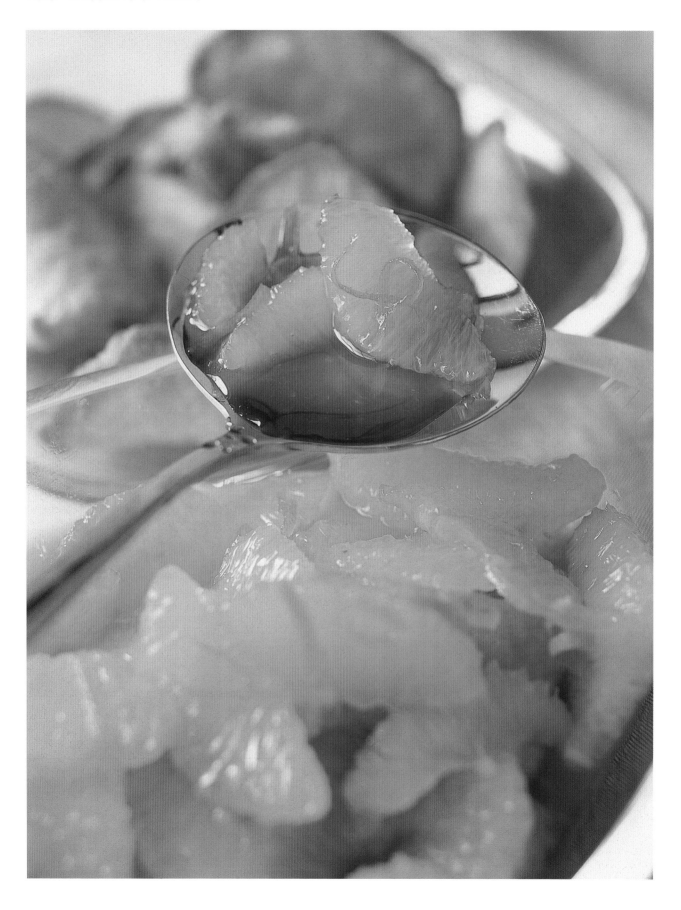

CARAMEL ORANGES WITH ALMOND & SESAME SEED COOKIES

Oranges are a useful source of calcium and also provide plenty of other vitamins and minerals, especially vitamin C. These cookies make a light, low-fat, tasty dessert.

1 Remove the zest from 3 of the oranges and set aside. To peel the oranges, slice them all across the top and bottom to reveal the flesh, then remove the skin and pith in strips by slicing downwards, following the shape of the orange.

2 Working over a bowl, remove the orange segments by slicing carefully between each segment and its membrane. Reserve the juice in the bowl. Put the orange segments to one side.

3 To make the orange caramel, put the sugar in a heavy-based saucepan with 3 tablespoons (45 ml) of water. Heat gently until the sugar dissolves, then bring to a rapid boil until it turns a rich, golden color.

4 Remove from the heat and carefully add the honey, the reserved orange juice and half the reserved orange zest. The caramel will form a blob on the bottom of the pan, so return to a gentle heat and dissolve in the juice. When the mixture is smooth, set aside to cool.

5 When cool, pour the caramel over the orange segments. Chill in the fridge until ready to serve.

6 Meanwhile, make the almond sesame cookies. Preheat the oven to 425°F (220°C). Beat the egg whites until stiff, then add the sugar and beat for 1 minute until the mixture is glossy. Using a metal spoon, fold in the flour, butter, sesame seeds, almonds, and the reserved orange zest.

7 Put teaspoons of the mixture onto a baking pan lined with baking parchment, about 2½ in (6 cm) apart. Bake for 5–6 minutes until golden, then remove from the oven. While the cookies are still warm, press them with a rolling pin to curve them—they will harden in seconds. If the cookies harden on the tray before shaping, return to the oven for a few minutes to soften.

8 To serve, remove the orange segments from the fridge and spoon into serving bowls. Serve with the almond sesame cookies.

FOR THE CARAMEL ORANGES

6 large oranges

1 cup (250 ml) superfine sugar

2 tablespoons (30 ml) liquid honey

FOR THE ALMOND SESAME COOKIES

2 egg whites

¾ cup (175 ml) superfine sugar

¾ cup (175 ml) all-purpose flour, sifted

¼ cup (50 ml) butter, melted

2 tablespoons (30 ml) sesame seeds

½ cup (125 ml) chopped, blanched almonds

Serves 6 (24 cookies)

¾ cup (175 ml) fresh blueberries

1 cup (250 ml) fresh raspberries

1 cup (250 ml) fresh strawberries, hulled and roughly chopped

Seeds and juice of 4 passion fruits

1¼ cups (300 ml) Balkan-style plain yogurt

¾ cup (175 ml) soft brown sugar

Serves 4

MIXED BERRY BRULÉE

This classic dish is made healthier by replacing the cream with lower-fat yogurt.

1 Mix the blueberries, raspberries, strawberries and passion fruit seeds and juice together in a large bowl and divide into 4 ovenproof ramekins.

2 Spoon the yogurt over the fruit and chill for at least 2 hours.

3 Remove the ramekins from the fridge and sprinkle the sugar over the yogurt. Place under a hot broiler until the sugar caramelizes, then serve immediately.

LEMON & PASSION FRUIT ROULADE

FOR THE MERINGUE

4 egg whites

1⅛ cups (260 ml) superfine sugar

1 level tablespoon (15 ml) cornstarch

2 teaspoons (10 ml) malt vinegar

1 teaspoon (5 ml) vanilla extract

FOR THE FILLING

4 tablespoons (60 ml) lemon curd

Seeds and juice of 4 passion fruits

¼ cup (50 ml) slivered almonds, toasted, to decorate

Confectioners' sugar, for dusting

1 cup (225 ml) Balkan-style plain yogurt

Serves 6

Yogurt contains considerably less fat than heavy cream and about three times more calcium, helping to make this a healthier alternative to more traditional cream-filled desserts.

1 Preheat the oven to 300°F (150°C). Line the base and sides of a 12½ × 8½ in (31.5 × 21.5 cm) jelly roll pan with nonstick baking parchment.

2 With an electric beater, beat the egg whites until they are frothy and have doubled in bulk, then gradually beat in the sugar until the mixture is very thick and shiny. Beat in the cornstarch, vinegar and vanilla extract.

3 Spoon the mixture into the prepared pan and level the surface. Bake for 50 minutes, or until the surface is just firm.

4 Meanwhile, to make the filling, mix together the lemon curd and passion fruit seeds and juice.

5 Remove the meringue from the oven and allow to cool for 10 minutes. Remove from pan and carefully peel off the paper. Lightly dust a sheet of baking parchment with toasted almonds and confectioners' sugar and place the meringue on the parchment. Spread the yogurt over the meringue, then drizzle the lemon and passion fruit mixture over the yogurt.

6 Using the parchment to help you, roll up the meringue from one of the long ends. Refrigerate for at least 30 minutes, or until ready to serve.

APRICOT RISOTTO

This dessert is a variation on traditional rice pudding—the fruity apricot coulis adds a healthy, modern twist.

1 Place the canned apricots in a blender or food processor and purée until smooth. Set to one side. Place the milk and sugar in a saucepan and gently heat, stirring occasionally, until the milk reaches simmering point. Reduce the heat and allow the milk to simmer.

2 Melt the butter in a large saucepan, add the rice and cook, stirring, for 1–2 minutes. Add the chopped apricots and cook for 1–2 minutes.

3 Add a ladle of the warm milk and cook, stirring continuously, until the liquid is absorbed. Continue adding the milk in the same way until all the milk is used and the rice is tender—this will take about 20 minutes.

4 Stir the puréed apricots into the rice, then spoon into bowls and decorate with toasted almonds.

14 oz (400 g) canned apricots in natural juice, drained

4 cups (1 liter) whole milk

2 tablespoons (30 ml) superfine sugar

1 tablespoon (15 ml) butter

¾ cup (175 ml) arborio rice

¾ cup (175 ml) dried apricots, roughly chopped

2 tablespoons (30 ml) slivered almonds, toasted

Serves 4

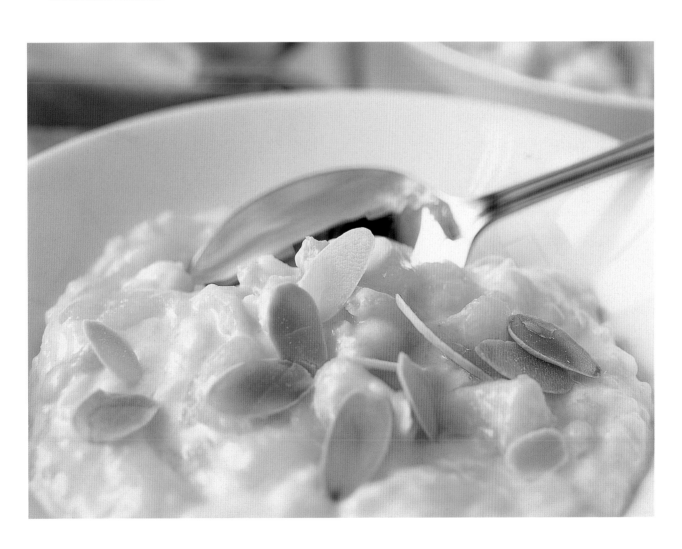

Frozen Strawberry Yogurt

1 lb (500 g) strawberries, hulled and roughly chopped

3 tablespoons (45 ml) apple juice

2 tablespoons (30 ml) crème de cassis (optional)

4 tablespoons (60 ml) confectioners' sugar

2 cups (500 ml) plain yogurt

Fresh fruit, to decorate

Serves 4

This is a healthy treat for a hot day. Although you can buy frozen yogurt in most supermarkets, if you have the time it is really worth making your own—once you've eaten homemade, store-bought will never taste quite the same. The frozen yogurt can be stored for up to 2 weeks in the freezer.

1 Place the strawberries in a saucepan. Add the apple juice and gently warm, stirring occasionally, until the strawberries become soft and pulpy.

2 Press the strawberries through a nylon sieve and collect their juice in a large bowl. Discard the seeds. Allow to cool completely, then beat in the crème de cassis (if using), sugar, and yogurt.

3 Pour the mixture into an ice-cream machine and churn until it becomes thick and frozen. If you don't have an ice-cream machine, transfer the mixture to a shallow freezer container. Freeze for at least 1 hour, or until the mixture begins to set around the edges. Remove the container from the freezer and beat the mixture until smooth, then return to the freezer. Freeze for another 30 minutes then beat again. Repeat the freezing and beating process two more times.

4 Transfer the frozen yogurt from the freezer to the fridge 20 minutes before serving. Decorate with fresh fruit to serve.

Lemon Mascarpone Ice Cream

1¼ lbs (500 g) mascarpone cheese

1 tablespoon (15 ml) lemon juice

Zest of 2 lemons

¾ cup (175 ml) confectioners' sugar

3 egg yolks

2 tablespoons (30 ml) orange liqueur

Fresh berries, to serve

Serves 6

This is an ideal dessert for a dinner party, especially when served with a selection of fresh summer berries. Remember that raw eggs are not suitable for the elderly, pregnant women, young children, or people who have immune deficiency disease.

1 Beat the mascarpone cheese, lemon juice and zest, confectioners' sugar, egg yolks, and orange-flavored liqueur together in a large bowl, until smooth.

2 Freeze the mixture in an ice cream machine, if you have one, or in a freezer container. If you use a freezer, beat the mixture at hourly intervals until the ice cream is frozen—this helps to prevent ice crystals forming and ensures an even-textured result.

3 Once frozen, remove the ice cream from the freezer and serve with fresh berries.

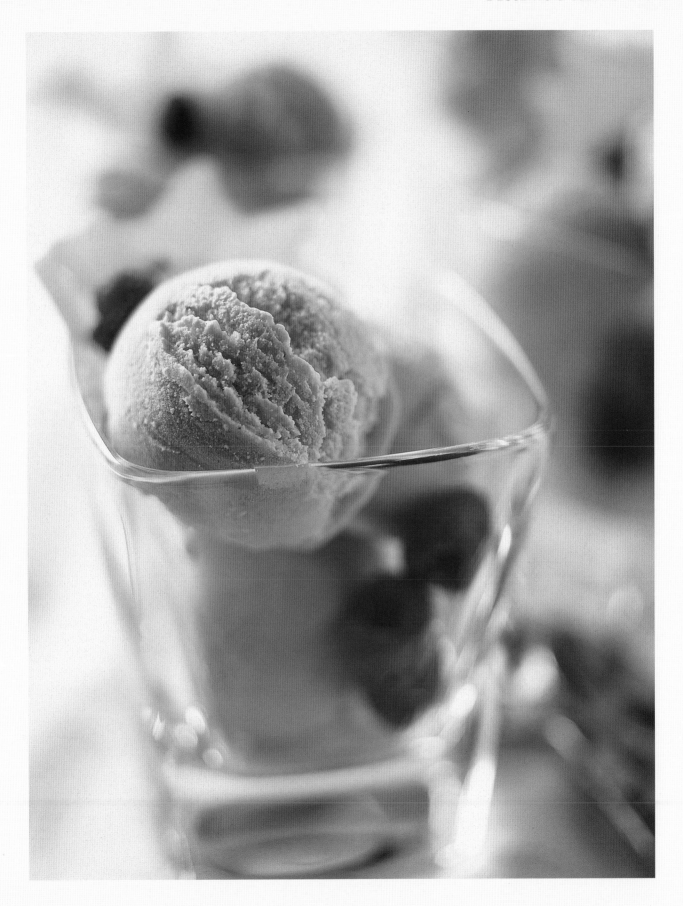

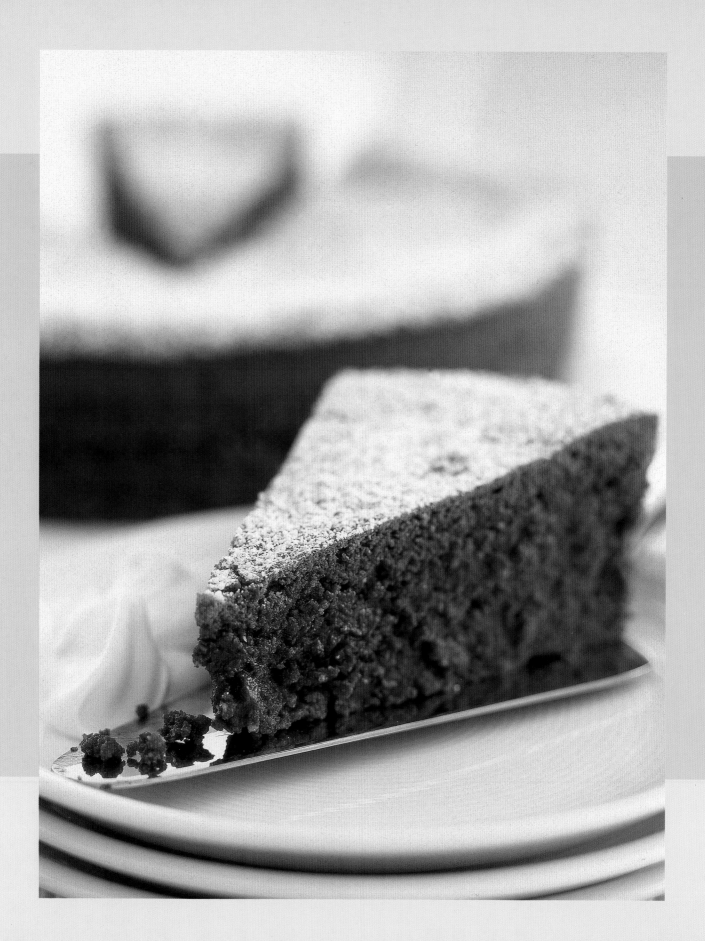

7 Home Baking

This chapter offers a selection of savory snacks, cookies and cakes that make delicious treats at any time of day. The recipes feature ingredients such as cheese, nuts, seeds, and fruit, which boost their calcium content, making them great for healthy bones.

SUN-DRIED TOMATO & PARMESAN CORN BREAD SQUARES

Serve this tasty bread with a bowl of steaming hot soup for a healthy and filling lunchtime snack.

1 large egg, beaten

1 cup (250 ml) plain yogurt

2 tablespoons (30 ml) butter, melted

1 cup (250 ml) fine cornmeal

3 tablespoons (45 ml) all-purpose flour

1 tablespoon (15 ml) baking powder

1 teaspoon (5 ml) chopped fresh rosemary

½ teaspoon (2 ml) salt

½ cup (125 ml) sun-dried tomatoes in oil roughly chopped

¾ cup (175 ml) drained, canned corn

½ cup (125 ml) Parmesan cheese, grated

Makes 9 squares

1 Preheat the oven to 350°F (180°C). Line the bottom of an 7 in (18 cm) square pan, approximately 1¼ in (3 cm) deep, with nonstick baking parchment.

2 Mix the egg, yogurt, and melted butter together. Stir in the cornmeal, flour, baking powder, rosemary, and salt. Add the sun-dried tomatoes, corn, and Parmesan and mix until thoroughly combined.

3 Turn the mixture into the prepared pan and bake for 30–40 minutes, or until a skewer inserted into the center of the loaf comes out clean.

4 Allow to cool in the pan for 10 minutes then turn out onto a cooling rack. When the bread is completely cold, cut into squares.

CHEESE & WATERCRESS SCONES

Light and easy to make, these scones make a delicious daytime snack. Watercress is an excellent source of vitamin C and vitamin E and provides substantial amounts of folic acid, niacin, and vitamin B_6.

2 cups (500 ml) sifted white pastry flour

1 teaspoon (5 ml) baking powder

¼ cup (50 ml) butter, diced

1¼ cups (300 ml) watercress, chopped with stalks removed

1¼ cups (300 ml) grated Gruyère cheese

Salt and pepper, to taste

7 tablespoons (105 ml) 2% milk, plus extra to glaze

Flour, for dusting

Makes 8 scones

1 Preheat the oven to 425°F (220°C). Place the flour and baking powder in a large bowl. Rub in the butter with your fingertips, until the mixture resembles fine bread crumbs.

2 Stir in the watercress, two-thirds of the cheese and the seasoning. Add the milk and stir to form a smooth, soft dough.

3 Turn the dough out on to a well-floured surface and roll out to ¾ in (2 cm) thick. Using a 3 in (7.5 cm) round cutter, cut out the scones. Press the trimmings together, re-roll, and cut out more scones, until all the dough has been used.

4 Place the scones on a greased baking pan. Brush the tops with milk, sprinkle over the remaining cheese, and bake for 10–15 minutes, or until golden brown. Transfer to a wire rack to cool.

PARMESAN & HERB TWISTS

These tasty little snacks are the perfect accompaniment for a glass of chilled white wine, and can also be served with dips or soups. They will keep for up to one week in an air-tight container.

1   Preheat the oven to 425°F (220°C). Dust the work surface and rolling pin with a little flour. Roll out the pastry until it is very thin, then trim into a neat rectangle or square. Cut in half.

2   Sprinkle one half of the pastry with an even layer of Parmesan cheese, chopped rosemary and thyme. Dampen the edges, then carefully place the other piece of pastry on top and gently press down.

3   Using a kitchen knife, cut the Parmesan and herb pastry into strips. Twist each strip around a few times, then place on a baking pan. Press the ends of the twists down so that they stick to the baking sheet—this stops them unwinding as they cook.

4   Bake the twists for about 10–12 minutes, or until golden brown, then remove the baking pan from the oven. Leave them on the baking pan for 5 minutes, then place on a wire rack to cool.

PESTO & PARMESAN TWISTS
Replace the rosemary and thyme with 3 tablespoons (45 ml) of green pesto (see recipe page 48). Spread the pesto over one half of the pastry and sprinkle with Parmesan. Then follow steps 3 and 4 as above.

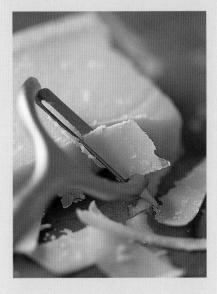

All-purpose flour, for dusting

---

1 lb 2 oz (500 g) ready-made puff pastry

¼ cup (50 ml) Parmesan cheese, grated

---

2 tablespoons (30 ml) fresh rosemary, chopped

---

1 tablespoon (15 ml) fresh thyme leaves, chopped

Makes about 24 twists

SODA BREAD

2½ cups (625 ml) whole-wheat flour

1½ cups (375 ml) steel-cut oats

2 teaspoons (10 ml) baking soda

1 teaspoon (5 ml) salt

1 teaspoon (5 ml) sugar

1¼ cups (300 ml) buttermilk

3–4 tablespoons (50–60 ml) 2% milk

Makes 1 loaf

This classic Irish recipe is extremely healthy and couldn't be easier to make. It's delicious served warm with slices of mature cheddar cheese.

1 Preheat the oven to 400°F (200°C). Place the flour, oats, baking soda, salt, and sugar in a large bowl. Make a well in the center and gradually beat in the buttermilk and enough milk to form a soft dough.

2 Knead the dough for 5 minutes, or until smooth. Shape into a round about 8 in (20 cm) in diameter. Using a sharp knife, cut a deep cross on the top of the dough. Place on a nonstick baking pan.

3 Bake for 30–45 minutes or until the bread sounds hollow when tapped on the bottom. Serve warm or leave to cool on a wire rack.

BANANA & PUMPKIN LOAF

7 tablespoons (105 ml) sunflower oil, plus extra for greasing

1 cup (250 ml) self-rising flour

½ cup (125 ml) whole-wheat flour

½ teaspoon (2 ml) baking soda

1 teaspoon (5 ml) ground cinnamon

¾ cup (175 ml) packed soft light brown sugar

4 tablespoons (60 ml) buttermilk or plain yogurt

2 eggs, beaten

2¼ cups (550 ml) canned or coarsely grated fresh pumpkin

1 medium banana, mashed

1 cup (250 ml) golden raisins

Makes 1 loaf

This moist fruity loaf is delicious served plain, but for a special treat, try adding the mascarpone topping on page 123.

1 Preheat the oven to 350°F (180°C). Lightly grease and line the base of a 9 x 5 in (22 x 12 cm) loaf pan with nonstick baking parchment.

2 Sift the flours, baking soda, and cinnamon into a large bowl. Stir in the sugar. Place the oil, buttermilk or yogurt, and eggs in a separate bowl and whisk to combine. Pour the liquid into the flour and beat with an electric beater for 1 minute.

3 Stir in the pumpkin, banana and golden raisins and transfer the mixture to the prepared pan. Bake for 1 hour, or until a skewer inserted into the middle comes out clean. Allow to cool in the pan for 5–10 minutes, then carefully transfer to a wire rack to cool completely.

SESAME OAT COOKIES

Sesame seeds are a good source of calcium and vitamin E and give these cookies a delicious nutty flavor.

1 Preheat the oven to 350°F (180°C). Lightly grease 2 cookie sheets.

2 Place the butter, syrup and sugar in a large saucepan. Heat the mixture gently, stirring occasionally, until the butter melts and the sugar dissolves.

3 Stir in the oats, sesame seeds, and flour and mix well.

4 Dissolve the baking soda in 1 teaspoon (5 ml) of hot water and stir into the mixture.

5 Allow the mixture to cool slightly, then roll into walnut-sized balls. Place on the prepared cookie sheets, allowing plenty of space for the mixture to spread as it bakes (you may need to cook the cookies in batches). Bake for 15 minutes, or until evenly browned.

6 Remove the cookies from the oven and leave on the cookie sheets to cool slightly. Using a palette knife, transfer to a wire rack to cool completely.

½ cup (125 ml) butter, plus extra for greasing

1 heaped tablespoon (20 ml) corn syrup

¾ cup (175 ml) light demerara (raw) sugar

¾ cup (175 ml) medium steel-cut or rolled oats

¼ cup (50 ml) sesame seeds

⅞ cup (200 ml) white all-purpose flour

1 teaspoon (5 ml) baking soda

Makes 26 cookies

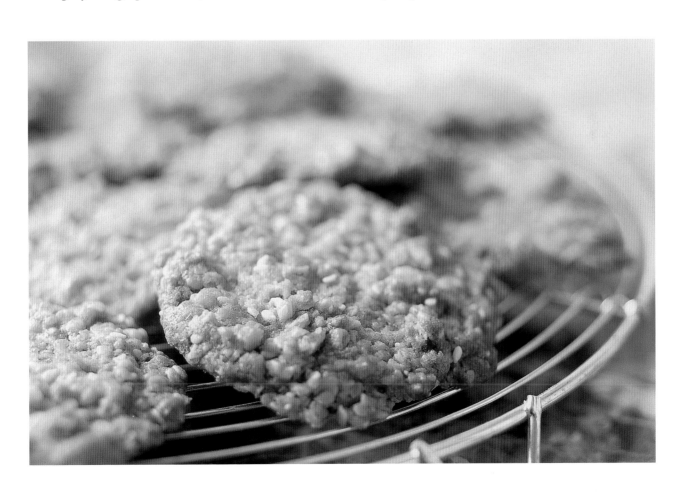

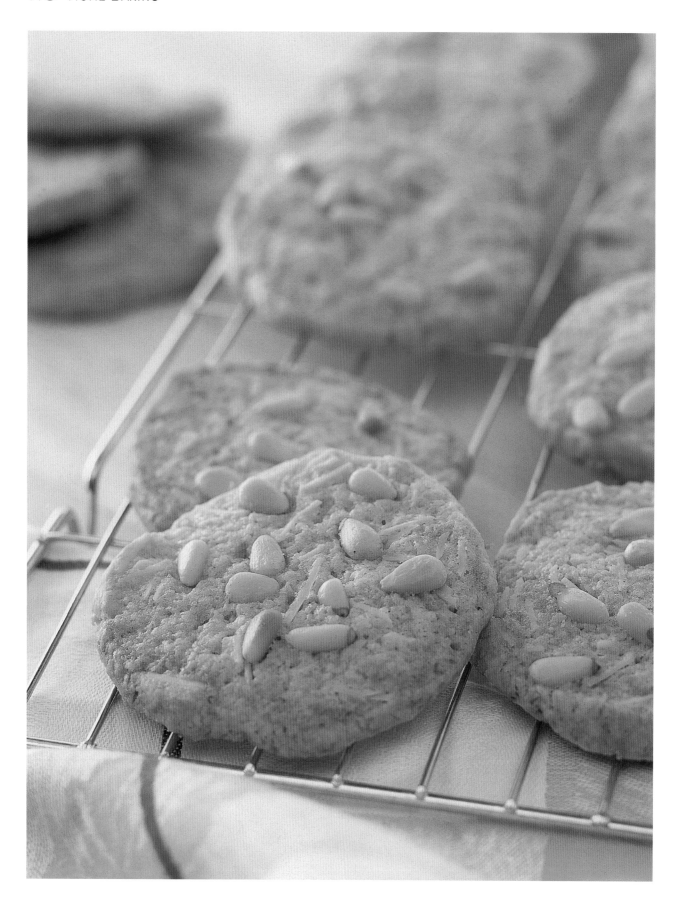

ALMOND & PINE NUT COOKIES

*Nuts are a good source of B vitamins and minerals, making
these cookies a healthy and tasty treat.*

1　Preheat the oven to 375˚F (190˚C). Lightly grease 2 cookie sheets.

2　Sift the flour and baking soda into a bowl. Add the butter and rub it in
with your fingertips until the mixture resembles fine bread crumbs. Add
the sugar and almonds, then stir in the egg, orange zest, and almond
extract and mix to a dough, adding a little milk if necessary.

3　Turn out onto a lightly floured surface and shape into a cylinder about 9 in
(23 cm) long. Cut into thin slices and place on the cookie sheets. Sprinkle
with the pine nuts, pressing them down lightly with your fingertips.

4　Bake the cookies for 8–10 minutes until pale golden (you may need to cook
them in batches). Allow to cool slightly before lifting them onto a wire
rack, then leave to cool completely.

APRICOT & PINE NUT COOKIES
Replace the almonds with ½ cup (125 ml) finely chopped, dried apricots. Follow
the recipe as above, omitting the almond extract.

1½ cups (375 ml) all-purpose flour,
plus extra for dusting

½ teaspoon (2 ml) baking soda

½ cup (125 ml) butter, diced

¾ cup (175 ml) brown sugar

¾ cup (175 ml) flaked almonds, roughly
chopped

---

1 egg, lightly beaten

Zest of 1 orange

Few drops almond extract

---

2 tablespoons (30 ml) milk

½ cup (125 ml) pine nuts, finely chopped

Makes 27 cookies

APRICOT & ORANGE MUFFINS

1¼ cups (300 ml) all-purpose flour

1½ teaspoons (7 ml) baking powder

½ teaspoon (2 ml) salt

2 tablespoons (30 ml) granulated sugar

2 tablespoons (30 ml) liquid honey

1 egg

⅓ cup (75 ml) orange juice

⅓ cup (75 ml) whole milk

¼ cup (50 ml) butter, melted and cooled

½ cup (125 ml) chopped dried apricots

Makes 6 muffins

These light-as-air muffins are studded with chewy apricots and orange zest. For a treat, they can also be served at breakfast.

1   Preheat the oven to 400°F (200°C). Line 6 deep muffin tins with paper cups.

2   Sift the flour, baking powder and salt into a large bowl. In another large bowl, mix together the sugar, honey, egg, orange juice, milk, and cooled butter. Sift the dry ingredients into the egg mixture and fold in gently with a metal spoon. Do not beat or stir the mixture.

3   Lightly fold in the chopped apricots. then divide the mixture equally into the paper cups. Bake for 15 minutes, or until well-risen and golden brown. A skewer inserted into the center of the muffins should come out clean. Leave in the tin for a few minutes, then transfer to a wire rack to cool. Serve warm or cold.

CITRUS YOGURT CAKE

1 cup (250 ml) yogurt

1¼ cups (300 ml) brown sugar

½ cup (125 ml) butter, melted, plus extra for greasing

3 eggs

Zest of ½ lemon, grated

Zest of ½ orange, grated

Zest of 1 lime, grated

2½ cups (600 ml) all-purpose flour

FOR THE MASCARPONE CREAM

9 oz (250 g) mascarpone cheese

1 tablespoon (15 ml) orange marmalade

Confectioners' sugar, for dusting

Serves 8

This moist citrus cake is made with plain yogurt and served with a lovely mascarpone cream. Another way to serve this cake is to split it in half and sandwich the two halves together with the mascarpone cream, then dredge the top with confectioners' sugar.

1   Preheat the oven to 350°F (180°C). Lightly grease an 8 in (20 cm) loose-bottomed shallow cake pan and line the base with parchment paper.

2   In a large bowl, whisk together the yogurt, sugar, melted butter, eggs, lemon, and orange and lime zest. Beat in the flour until well mixed.

3   Pour the cake mixture into the prepared pan and bake in the center of the oven for 60–70 minutes, or until a skewer inserted into the center of the cake comes out clean. Leave to cool for 10 minutes, then transfer to a cake rack to cool completely.

4   Meanwhile, beat the mascarpone with the marmalade. Cover and chill until ready to use.

5   Dust the top of the cake with confectioners' sugar. Cut into wedges and serve with a spoonful of the mascarpone cream.

LEMON & POPPY SEED DRIZZLE LOAF CAKE

Poppy seeds are a useful source of calcium, particularly for people on dairy-free diets. This cake is good on its own or with a spoonful of crème fraîche or yogurt.

1 Preheat the oven to 350°F (180°C). Grease and line a loaf pan.

2 Place the butter or margarine, sugar, eggs, flour, baking powder, salt, lemon zest, and juice into a food processor and process until smooth. Fold in the poppy seeds.

3 Spoon the mixture into the prepared pan and level the surface. Bake for 50–55 minutes, or until well risen and firm to the touch. Turn out and cool on a wire rack.

4 For the topping, mix the sugar with enough lemon juice to form a smooth consistency. Drizzle over the top of the cake and decorate with the shredded candied lemon peel.

FOR THE CAKE

1 cup (250 ml) butter or margarine

1¼ cups (300 ml) brown sugar

3 eggs

2½ cups (600 ml) whole-wheat flour

1 teaspoon (5 ml) baking powder

Pinch salt

Zest and juice of 2 large lemons

½ cup (125 ml) poppy seeds

FOR THE TOPPING

½ cup (125 ml) confectioners' sugar

2–3 teaspoons (10–15 ml) lemon juice

Candied lemon peel, shredded, to decorate

Makes 1 loaf

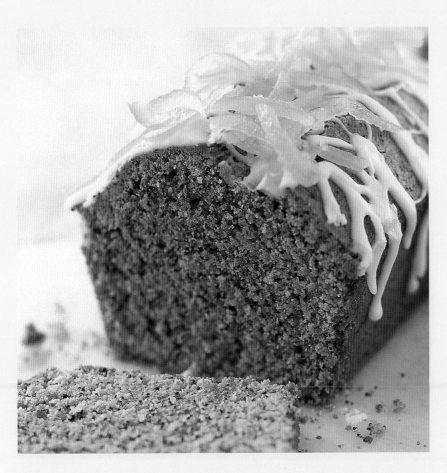

RICH CHOCOLATE CAKE

7 oz (200 g) dark chocolate (about 70% cocoa)

2 teaspoons (10 ml) dry instant coffee

1 cup (250 ml) unsalted butter, softened

1 cup (250 ml) superfine sugar

4 eggs, separated

1¼ cups (300 ml) ground almonds

½ cup (125 ml) cornstarch

Confectioners' sugar, for dusting

Crème fraîche, to serve

Serves 10

Everyone's favorite treat, this moist, rich chocolate cake not only tastes fantastic but, thanks to the ground almonds, is also a good source of calcium. Serve with yogurt or low-fat crème fraîche.

1   Preheat the oven to 350°F (180°C). Lightly grease an 8 in (20 cm) loose-bottomed cake pan and line the base with parchment paper.

2   Place the chocolate and coffee in a bowl over a pan of simmering water and melt. In a large bowl, cream the butter and sugar until pale and fluffy. Beat in the eggs yolks, one at a time, then stir in the chocolate and coffee mixture, almonds, and cornstarch.

3   In a large, clean bowl, beat the egg whites until they form soft peaks. Fold a quarter of the beaten egg whites into the chocolate mixture to loosen it, then gradually fold in the remainder. Pour the mixture into the prepared pan and bake for 50–60 minutes, or until it springs back when touched. Cover the cake with baking parchment after 50 minutes. Allow to cool completely before carefully removing it from the pan.

4   Cut the cake into wedges, dust with a little confectioners' sugar, and serve with crème fraîche or other cream topping, if liked.

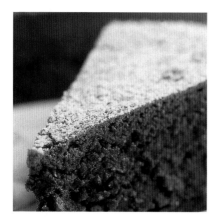

FOR THE CARROT CAKE

Butter, for greasing

Flour, for dusting

1 cup (250 ml) unsalted butter or margarine, softened

1⅛ cups (260 ml) brown sugar

1¼ cups (300 ml) white pastry flour

1 teaspoon (5 ml) baking powder

½ teaspoon (2 ml) ground allspice

4 eggs

Zest of 1 large orange

CARROT CAKE WITH MASCARPONE TOPPING

This cake is guaranteed to be a hit with both children and adults. The mascarpone cheese makes a deliciously rich and creamy frosting.

1   Preheat the oven to 350°F (180°C). Grease two 8 in (20 cm) layer pans. Dust the sides of the pans with flour and shake out the excess.

2   Cream the butter or margarine and sugar together in a bowl until pale and fluffy. Sift the flour, baking powder, and allspice into the bowl. Add the eggs, orange rind and juice, and ground almonds and beat well, then stir in the walnuts and the carrots.

3   Divide the mixture equally between the two pans and level the surface. Bake for 35–40 minutes until the cakes have risen and are firm to the touch. Leave in the pans for 5 minutes, then transfer to a wire rack to cool.

4　For the topping, beat the mascarpone cheese and sugar together in a bowl until smooth. Spread half the mixture between the layers, then spread the remaining mixture over the top of the cake. Arrange the walnut halves around the edge of the cake to decorate.

ORANGE MASCARPONE TOPPING
Beat together 1¼ lb (500 g) mascarpone cheese with 1 teaspoon (5 ml) orange zest, 2 tablespoons (30 ml) orange juice, and 2 tablespoons (30 ml) confectioners' sugar. Use to spread between the layers, and spread the remainder over the top of the cake. Decorate with walnuts and orange zest.

1 tablespoon (15 ml) orange juice

½ cup (125 ml) ground almonds

1 cup (250 ml) finely grated carrots

1¼ cups (300 ml) coarsely chopped walnuts

FOR THE MASCARPONE TOPPING

1¼ lb (500 g) mascarpone cheese

2 tablespoons (30 ml) confectioners' sugar

½ cup (125 ml) walnut halves, to decorate

Serves 8–10

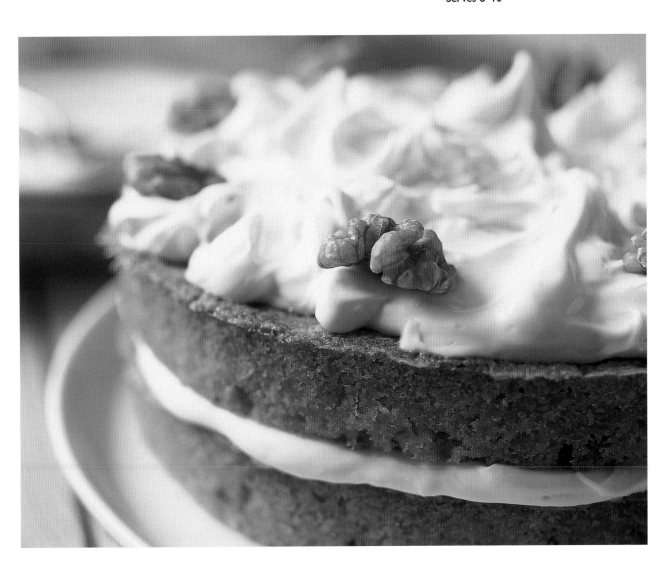

The nutritional information for each recipe refers to a single serving, unless otherwise stated. Optional ingredients are not included. The figures are intended as a guide only. If salt is given in a measured amount in the recipe, it has been included in the analysis; if the recipe suggests adding a pinch of salt or seasoning to taste, salt has not been included.

p.12 Sweet Fruit Oatmeal
calories 235; KJ 996; protein 6g; fat 4g; saturated fat 1g; fiber 3g; sodium 50mg; calcium 75mg

p.12 Apple & Blueberry Granola
calories 460–306; KJ 1944–1296; protein 15–10g; fat 13–9g; saturated fat 1g; fiber 7.5–5g; sodium 127–85mg; calcium 330–220mg

p.13 Spiced Fruit Compote
calories 340; KJ 1452; protein 7g; fat 9g; saturated fat 3g; fiber 5g; sodium 293mg; calcium 143mg

p.14 Dried Fruit Spread
calories 40; KJ 152; protein 1g; fat 0g; saturated fat 0g; fiber 1g; sodium 6mg; calcium 25mg

p.14 Bagels with Raspberries & Ricotta
calories 300; KJ 1220; protein 12g; fat 6g; saturated fat 3g; fiber 3g; sodium 40mg; calcium 100mg

p.14 Banana & Almond Smoothie
calories 320; KJ 1350; protein 13g; fat 15g; saturated fat 4g; fiber 3g; sodium 128mg; calcium 325mg

p.15 Apricot & Orange Smoothie
calories 170; KJ 727; protein 3g; fat 1g; saturated fat 0g; fiber 4g; sodium 29mg; calcium 65mg

p.15 Strawberry Smoothie
calories 100; KJ 410; protein 6g; fat 3g; saturated fat 0.5g; fiber 2g; sodium 60mg; calcium 70mg

p.17 Cheesy Scrambled Eggs
calories 300; KJ 1270; protein 22g; fat 23g; saturated fat 10g; fiber 0g; sodium 365mg; calcium 268mg

p.17 Smoked Haddock Omelet
calories 390; KJ 1629; protein 36g; fat 27g; saturated fat 12g; fiber 0g; sodium 1136mg; calcium 317mg

p.18 Boiled Eggs with Sour Cream & Smoked Salmon
calories 310; KJ 1295; protein 19g; fat 18g; saturated fat 8g; fiber 1g; sodium 779mg; calcium 113mg

p.19 Smoked Haddock & Corn Fritters
calories 244; KJ 1036; protein 17g; fat 5g; saturated fat 1g; fiber 3g; sodium 733mg; calcium 128mg

p.19 Stuffed Mushrooms
calories 400; KJ 1199; protein 24g; fat 11g; saturated fat 3g; fiber 4.5g; sodium 1199mg; calcium 250mg

p.22 Broccoli & Stilton Soup
calories 275; KJ 1148; protein 16g; fat 16g; saturated fat 8g; fiber 4g; sodium 525mg; calcium 265mg

p.22 Moroccan Spiced Chickpea Soup
calories 210; KJ 876; protein 10g; fat 9g; saturated fat 1g; fiber 6g; sodium 440mg; calcium 90mg

p.23 Roasted Red Pepper Soup with Feta & Basil
calories 140; KJ 580; protein 5g; fat 8g; saturated fat 3g; fiber 3g; sodium 392mg; calcium 90mg

p.25 French Onion Soup
calories 370; KJ 1547; protein 13g; fat 18g; saturated fat 10g; fiber 3g; sodium 869mg; calcium 288mg

p.25 Garden Pea & Watercress Soup with Sesame Croûtons
calories 380; KJ 1605; protein 12g; fat 27g; saturated fat 7g; fiber 7g; sodium 545mg; calcium 118mg

p.26 Smoked Haddock & Corn Chowder
calories 390; KJ 1638; protein 35g; fat 9g; saturated fat 5g; fiber 3g; sodium 1865mg; calcium 205mg

p.26 Baked Ricotta with Roasted Vine Tomatoes
calories 350; KJ 14560; protein 24g; fat 26g; saturated fat 14g; fiber 1g; sodium 484mg; calcium 578mg

p.27 Mushroom & Goat Cheese in Eggplant Parcels
calories 260; KJ 1062; protein 11g; fat 22g; saturated fat 8g; fiber 4g; sodium 301mg; calcium 144mg

p.28 Cherry Tomato & Goat Cheese Tartlets
calories 440; KJ 1838; protein 13g; fat 32g; saturated fat 10g; fiber 0.5g; sodium 398mg; calcium 200mg

p.28 Tomato & Mozzarella Salad
calories 390; KJ 1622; protein 20g; fat 33g; saturated fat 12g; fiber 1.5g; sodium 471mg; calcium 453mg

p.29 Watercress, Pear, & Roquefort Salad
calories 425; KJ 1763; protein 14g; fat 37g; saturated fat 13g; fiber 3g; sodium 857mg; calcium 367mg

p.29 Avocado & Smoked Salmon Rolls
calories 350; KJ 1476; protein 25g; fat 27g; saturated fat 10g; fiber 2g; sodium 1473mg; calcium 140mg

p.30 Roasted Red Pepper Dip
calories 135–90; KJ 570–380; protein 18–12g; fat 1–4.5g; saturated fat 0g; fiber 2–1g; sodium 188–125mg; calcium 150–100mg

p.30 Tzatziki
calories 125–83; KJ 512–341; protein 7–5g; fat 9–6g; saturated fat 5–3.5g; fiber 0.5g; sodium 74–50mg; calcium 166–111mg

p.30 Creamy Guacamole
calories 200; KJ 892; protein 3g; fat 21g; saturated fat 5g; fiber 4g; sodium 21mg; calcium 40mg

p.34 Hummus
calories 275; KJ 1144; protein 9g; fat 21g; saturated fat 3g; fiber 5g; sodium 196mg; calcium 140mg

p.34 Red Pepper Hummus
calories 280; KJ 1184; protein 10g; fat 19g; saturated fat 3g; fiber 6g; sodium 196mg; calcium 122mg

p.35 Falafel with Salad in Pita
calories 485; KJ 2050; protein 20g; fat 12g; saturated fat 1g; fiber 6g; sodium 905mg; calcium 205mg

p.36 Quick Ciabatta Pizza
calories 300; KJ 1241; protein 11g; fat 15g; saturated fat 5g; fiber 2g; sodium 440mg; calcium 130mg

p.36 Croque Monsieur
calories 555; KJ 2341; protein 23g; fat 36g; saturated fat 19g; fiber 1g; sodium 1012mg; calcium 554mg

p.38 Peppered Smoked Mackerel Spread
calories 342; KJ 1419; protein 19g; fat 29g; saturated fat 9g; fiber 0g; sodium 751mg; calcium 110mg

p.38 Chicken Tikka Salad
calories 290; KJ 1205; protein 29g; fat 18g; saturated fat 4g; fiber 1g; sodium 177mg; calcium 70mg

p.39 Chicken Caesar Salad with Parmesan Crisps
calories 425; KJ 1775; protein 38g; fat 23g; saturated fat 6g; fiber 1g; sodium 593mg; calcium 280mg

p.40 Feta Omelet with Arugula & Red Pepper
calories 500; KJ 2095; protein 28g; fat 41g; saturated fat 19g; fiber 1.5g; sodium 1315mg; calcium 356mg

p.40 Twice Baked Goat Cheese Soufflés
calories 210; KJ 875; protein 9g; fat 16g; saturated fat 10g; fiber 0g; sodium 343mg; calcium 225mg

p.42 Spinach & Roquefort Crêpes
calories 430; KJ 1796; protein 22g; fat 25g; saturated fat 13g; fiber 4g; sodium 1294mg; calcium 654mg

p.42 Cajun Cheese Potato Skins with Tomato & Red Onion Salad
calories 300; KJ 1271; protein 12g; fat 14g; saturated fat 7g; fiber 2g; sodium 223mg; calcium 235mg

p.44 Bacon & Ricotta Tart
calories 400; KJ 1676; protein 18g; fat 20g; saturated fat 10g; fiber 2g; sodium 1255mg; calcium 229mg

p.45 Sweet Potato with Cottage Cheese & Crispy Bacon
calories 390; KJ 1652; protein 27g; fat 8g; saturated fat 4g; fiber 6g; sodium 1415mg; calcium 138mg

p.45 Spinach & Potato Cake
calories 420; KJ 1750; protein 18g; fat 24g; saturated fat 13g; fiber 4g; sodium 330mg; calcium 366g

p.48 Brie-stuffed Chicken with Creamy Pesto
calories 460; KJ 1931; protein 47g; fat 28g; saturated fat 13g; fiber 0g; sodium 937mg; calcium 300mg

p.49 Chicken & Wild Mushroom Stroganoff
calories 380; KJ 1568; protein 35g; fat 22g; saturated fat 10g; fiber 2g; sodium 388mg; calcium 27mg

p.49 Garlic Chicken in Yogurt
calories 440; KJ 1813; protein 29g; fat 34g; saturated fat 8g; fiber 2g; sodium 173mg; calcium 200mg

p.50 Coronation Chicken Salad
calories 760–506; KJ 3158–2105; protein 40–27g; fat 52–35g; saturated fat 15–10g; fiber 3–2g; sodium 565–376mg; calcium 115–77mg

p 51 Chicken & Sesame Bites
calories 300; KJ 1248; protein 23g; fat 17g; saturated fat 3g; fiber 2g; sodium 228mg; calcium 166mg

p.51 Quick Turkey Cassoulet
calories 560; KJ 2374; protein 58g; fat 15g; saturated fat 5g; fiber 12g; sodium 2318mg; calcium 336mg

p.52 Pork Stuffed with Apricots & Pine Nuts
calories 555–370; KJ 2320–1547; protein 53–35g; fat 29–19g; saturated fat 8–5g; fiber 2–1g; sodium 525–350mg; calcium 85–57mg

p.54 Pork with Bok Choy & Black Bean Sauce
calories 540; KJ 2273; protein 37g; fat 22g; saturated fat 5g; fiber 5g; sodium 1785mg; calcium 190mg

p.54 Pork Escalopes with Celeriac Cream Mash
calories 5116; KJ 2153; protein 31g; fat 29g; saturated fat 6g; fiber 6g; sodium 348mg; calcium 88mg

p.56 Polenta with Bacon & Mushrooms
calories 480; KJ 2000; protein 32g; fat 24g; saturated fat 11g; fiber 2g; sodium 1622mg; calcium 431mg

p.57 Broccoli & Smoked Ham Tagliatelle
calories 850; KJ 3557; protein 33g; fat 48g; saturated fat 29g; fiber 9g; sodium 1033mg; calcium 369mg

p.58 Skewered Lamb with Tomato, Chili & Yogurt Marinade
calories 600; KJ 2500; protein 43g; fat 24g; saturated fat 8g; fiber 0g; sodium 275mg; calcium 75mg

p.59 Garlic & Cumin Roasted Lamb with Apricot & Chickpea Salsa
calories 460; KJ 1919; protein 42g; fat 22g; saturated fat 8g; fiber 5g; sodium 334mg; calcium 70mg

p.60 Moroccan Lamb with Chickpeas & Apricots
calories 440; KJ 1841; protein 32g; fat 15g; saturated fat 5g; fiber 6g; sodium 492mg; calcium 90mg

p.61 Moussaka
calories 540; KJ 2241; protein 43g; fat 31g; saturated fat 14g; fiber 4g; sodium 460mg; calcium 424mg

p.62 Shepherd's Pie
calories 510; KJ 2142; protein 35g; fat 23g; saturated fat 12g; fiber 5g; sodium 344mg; calcium 210mg

p.62 Blue Cheese & Walnut Steaks
calories 480; KJ 2000; protein 45g; fat 33g; saturated fat 14g; fiber 0g; sodium 488mg; calcium 125mg

p.63 Meatballs with Mozzarella & Tomato Sauce
calories 470; KJ 1964; protein 38g; fat 24g; saturated fat 10g; fiber 2g; sodium 505mg; calcium 271mg

p.65 Ground Beef with Polenta Topping
calories 630; KJ 2612; protein 39g; fat 34g; saturated fat 12g; fiber 3g; sodium 666mg; calcium 311mg

p.66 Salmon Fish Cakes
calories 540; KJ 2260; protein 29g; fat 27g; saturated fat 4g; fiber 12g; sodium 850mg; calcium 367mg

p.66 Salmon & Leek Lasagna
calories 590; KJ 2454; protein 37g; fat 34g; saturated fat 18g; fiber 2g; sodium 744mg; calcium 785mg

p.67 Smoked Salmon & Dill Quiche
calories 500; KJ 2090; protein 13g; fat 41g; saturated fat 21g; fiber 1g; sodium 718mg; calcium 140mg

p.68 Quick Salmon Kedgeree
calories 420; KJ 1741; protein 23g; fat 16g; saturated fat 6g; fiber 0g; sodium 303mg; calcium 206mg

p.68 Salmon with a Crumb Crust
calories 380; KJ 1590; protein 30g; fat 25g; carbohydrate 10g; fiber 0g; sodium 382mg; calcium 200mg

p.69 Cod & Broccoli Cheese Pie
calories 894; KJ 3712; protein 39g; fat 65g; saturated fat 41g; fiber 4g; sodium 617mg; calcium 394mg

p.70 Cod Baked in Yogurt
calories 160; KJ 680; protein 34g; fat 1.5g; saturated fat 0g; fiber 0g; sodium 258mg; calcium 87mg

p.70 Poached Haddock with Spinach & Poached Egg
calories 270; KJ 1147; protein 42g; fat 10g; saturated fat 3g; fiber 3g; sodium 1423mg; calcium 350mg

p.71 Fish Pie with Rösti Topping
calories 615; KJ 2552; protein 22g; fat 46g; saturated fat 28g; fiber 3g; sodium 891mg; calcium 123mg

p.71 Deep-fried Smelt
calories 550; KJ 2299; protein 16g; fat 52g; saturated fat 6g; fiber 0g; sodium 278mg; calcium 711mg

p.72 Monkfish Kabobs with Roasted Vegetables & Pesto
calories 480; KJ 2000; protein 31g; fat 35g; saturated fat 8g; fiber 4g; sodium 523mg; calcium 240mg

p.73 Grilled Swordfish with Salsa Verde
calories 330; KJ 1358; protein 36g; fat 23g; saturated fat 4g; fiber 0g; sodium 365mg; calcium 45mg

p.74 Shrimp & Spinach Roulade
calories 400; KJ 1636; protein 15g; fat 33g; saturated fat 19g; fiber 1g; sodium 895mg; calcium 218mg

p.74 Penne with Shrimp & Asparagus
calories 680; KJ 2864; protein 42g; fat 33g; saturated fat 8g; fiber 3g; sodium 1844mg; calcium 456mg

p.76 Warm Lentil & Feta Salad
calories 404; KJ 1691; protein 22g; fat 22g; saturated fat 9g; fiber 6g; sodium 734mg; calcium 225mg

p.77 Spiced Spinach Lentil & Feta Phyllo Pie
calories 481; KJ 2000; protein 22g; fat 11g; saturated fat 5g; fiber 6g; sodium 682mg; calcium 306mg

p.78 Cheese & Leek Sausages
calories 372; KJ 1552; protein 14g; fat 24g; saturated fat 8g; fiber 1g; sodium 405mg; calcium 255mg

p.78 Vegetable Patties
calories 507; KJ 2117; protein 23g; fat 2g; saturated fat 13g; fiber 4g; sodium 575mg; calcium 500mg

p.79 Spiced Tofu Burgers
calories 160; KJ 669; protein 8g; fat 9g; saturated fat 1g; fiber 2g; sodium 85mg; calcium 322mg

p.80 Roasted Thai-style Tofu with Stir-fried Vegetables
calories 290; KJ 1208; protein 15g; fat 17g; saturated fat 2g; fiber 5g; sodium 986mg; calcium 681mg

p.82 Marinated Tofu with Satay Sauce
calories 452; KJ 1877; protein 19g; fat 36g; saturated fat 7g; fiber 3g; sodium 772mg; calcium 348mg

p.83 Hot Spiced Chickpeas
calories 175; KJ 741; protein 9g; fat 5g; saturated fat 0.6g; fiber 6g; sodium 264mg; calcium 64mg

p.83 Chickpea & Potato Stew
calories 393; KJ 1654; protein 17g; fat 12g; saturated fat 1g; fiber 10g; sodium 693mg; calcium 149mg

p.84 Mixed Beans with a Cornmeal Topping
calories 544; KJ 2290; protein 30g; fat 18g; saturated fat 8g; fiber 13g; sodium 1955mg; calcium 438mg

p.85 Butternut Squash &
Gruyère Risotto
calories 537; KJ 2230; protein 17g;
fat 30g; saturated fat 13g;
fiber 3g; sodium 399mg;
calcium 373mg

p.87 Roasted Vegetable Lasagna
calories 473; KJ 1986; protein 25g;
fat 23g; saturated fat 11g;
fiber 5g; sodium 423mg;
calcium 505mg

p.87 Pappardelle with Spicy
Tomato Sauce & Ricotta
calories 392; KJ 1659; protein 15g;
fat 10g; saturated fat 4g; fiber 4g;
sodium 149mg; calcium 177mg

p.88 Broccoli & Gruyère Soufflé
calories 245; KJ 1016; protein 13g;
fat 18g; saturated fat 10g;
fiber 1g; sodium 259mg;
calcium 286mg

p.89 Mediterranean Stuffed
Peppers with Couscous
calories 434; KJ 1802; protein 14g;
fat 26g; saturated fat 7g;
fiber 3.2g; sodium 864mg;
calcium 160mg

p.92 Green Beans with Feta &
Sun-dried Tomatoes
calories 125; KJ 511; protein 4g;
fat 10g; saturated fat 3g; fiber 1g;
sodium 400mg; calcium 95mg

p.92 Roasted Baby Carrots with
Parmesan & Cilantro Topping
calories 160; KJ 670; protein 6g;
fat 10g; saturated fat 15g;
fiber 3g; sodium 202mg;
calcium 188mg

p.93 Asian-style Broccoli
calories 75; KJ 310; protein 5g; fat
5g; saturated fat 1g; fiber 3g;
sodium 224mg; calcium 72mg

p.94 Honeyed Parsnips with
Sesame Seeds
calories 250; KJ 1069; protein 4g;
fat 14g; saturated fat 7g;
fiber 8g; sodium 113mg;
calcium 125mg

p.95 Fantail Roast Potatoes with
Sesame Seeds
calories 304; KJ 1218; protein 7g;
fat 9g; saturated fat 1g; fiber 4g;
sodium 22mg; calcium 50mg

p.96 Sweet Potato & Anchovy
Gratin
calories 650; KJ 2707; protein 14g;
fat 50g; saturated fat 29g;
fiber 4g; sodium 610mg;
calcium 321mg

p.96 Eggplant & Tomato Gratin
calories 334; KJ 1384; protein 9g;
fat 31g; saturated fat16g; fiber 2g;
sodium 273mg; calcium 186mg

p.98 Cauliflower & Broccoli
Cheese
calories 520; KJ 2167; protein 13g;
fat 48g; saturated fat 29g;
fiber 3g; sodium 457mg;
calcium 296mg

p.98 Apple, Walnut, &
Watercress Salad
calories 223; KJ 936; protein 3g;
fat 20g; saturated fat 2g; fiber 2g;
sodium 15mg; calcium 63mg

p.99 Potato Salad with Blue
Cheese Dressing
calories 250; KJ 1039; protein 11g;
fat 13g; saturated fat 8g;
fiber 2g; sodium 311mg;
calcium 136mg

p.102 Fudgy Nut Pie
calories 615; KJ 2580; protein 8g;
fat 32g; saturated fat 12g;
fiber 2g; sodium 470mg;
calcium 75mg

p.102 Spiced Apple & Raisin
Crêpes
calories 338; KJ 1434; protein 8g;
fat 5g; saturated fat 1.5g; fiber 4g;
sodium 172mg; calcium 155mg

p.103 Rich Chocolate & Fig
Puddings with Chocolate Sauce
calories 6240; KJ 2612; protein
10g; fat 33g; saturated fat 19g;
fiber 2g; sodium 477mg; calcium
156mg

p.104 Dates Stuffed with Ricotta
calories 180; KJ 766; protein 4g;
fat 5g; saturated fat 2g; fiber 1.5g;
sodium 53mg; calcium 82mg

p.104 Brandied Prunes with
Yogurt
calories 149; KJ 629; protein 3g;
fat 3g; saturated fat 2g; fiber 2g;
sodium 33mg; calcium 67mg

p.105 Lemon & Strawberry
Cheesecake
calories 800–600; KJ 3342–2507;
protein 8–6g; fat 57–43g;
saturated fat 34–26g;
fiber 2–1.5g; sodium 560–419mg;
calcium 206–154mg

p.107 Caramel Oranges with
Almond & Sesame Seed
Cookies
calories 455; KJ 1921; protein 6g;
fat 14g; saturated fat 5g; fiber 3g;
sodium 92mg; calcium 123mg

p.108 Mixed Berry Brulée
calories 240; KJ 1011; protein 6g;
fat 7g; saturated fat 4g;
fiber 1.5g; sodium 62mg;
calcium 130mg

p.108 Lemon & Passion Fruit
Roulade
calories 350; KJ 1465; protein 6g;
fat 15g; saturated fat 8g;
fiber 1g; sodium 84mg;
calcium 80mg

p.109 Apricot Risotto
calories 480; KJ 1996; protein 14g;
fat 17g; saturated fat 8g;
fiber 3g; sodium 175mg;
calcium 353mg

p.110 Frozen Strawberry Yogurt
calories 241; KJ 1008; protein 9g;
fat 11.5g; saturated fat 6g;
fiber 1g; sodium 100mg;
calcium 210mg

p.110 Lemon Mascarpone
Ice Cream
calories 490; KJ 2037; protein 4g;
fat 42g; saturated fat 25g;
fiber 0g; sodium 258mg;
calcium 94mg

p.114 Sun-dried Tomato &
Parmesan Corn Bread Squares
calories 200; KJ 830; protein 7g;
fat 10g; saturated fat 4g; fiber
0.5g; sodium 504mg;
calcium 130mg

p.114 Cheese & Watercress
Scones
calories 240; KJ 1025; protein 8g;
fat 11g; saturated fat 7g;
fiber 1g; sodium 375mg;
calcium 329mg

p.115 Parmesan & Herb Twists
calories 80; KJ 330; protein 1g;
fat 5g; saturated fat 0.5g;
fiber 0g; sodium 73mg;
calcium 24mg

p.116 Soda Bread
(per slice) calories 174; KJ 741;
protein 7g; fat 2g; saturated fat
0g; fiber 4g; sodium 493mg;
calcium 64mg

p.116 Banana & Pumpkin Loaf
(per slice) calories 240; KJ 1004;
protein 4g; fat 9g; saturated fat
1g; fiber 2g; sodium 137mg;
calcium 77mg

p.117 Sesame Oat Cookies
calories 100; KJ 415; protein 1g;
fat 6g; saturated fat 2g;
fiber 0.5g; sodium 95mg;
calcium 22mg

p.119 Almond & Pine Nut
Cookies
calories 111; KJ 462; protein 2g;
fat 7g; saturated fat 3g;
fiber 0.5g; sodium 64mg;
calcium 22mg

p.120 Apricot & Orange Muffins
calories 245; KJ 1031; protein 5g;
fat 9g; saturated fat 5g; fiber 1g;
sodium 365mg; calcium 90mg

p.120 Citrus Yogurt Cake
calories 565; KJ 2365; protein 9g;
fat 31g; saturated fat 18g;
fiber 1.5g; sodium 266mg;
calcium 156mg

p.121 Lemon & Poppy Seed
Drizzle Loaf Cake
calories 335; KJ 1399; protein 6g;
fat 19g; saturated fat 11g; fiber 3g;
sodium 254mg; calcium 94mg

p.122 Rich Chocolate Cake
calories 520; KJ 2155; protein 8g;
fat 36g; saturated fat 16g;
fiber 1.5g; sodium 193mg;
calcium 80mg

p.122 Carrot Cake with
Mascarpone Topping
calories 747; KJ 3103; protein 10g;
fat 60g; saturated fat 29g;
fiber 2g; sodium 427mg;
calcium 131mg

Index

ACKNOWLEDGEMENTS

Editorial assistance: Tom Broder
Nutritional analysis: Fiona Hunter
Production: Nigel Reed
IT: Paul Stradling